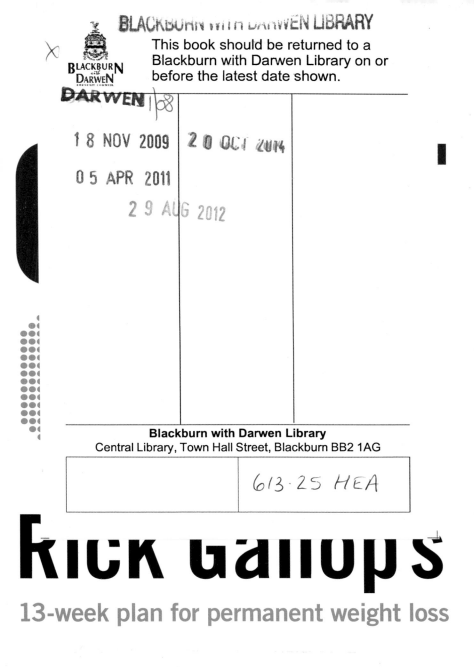
Rick Gallop's

13-week plan for permanent weight loss

D0795450

First published in Great Britain in 2008 by
Virgin Books Ltd
Thames Wharf Studios
Rainville Road
London
W6 9HA

Published by arrangement with Random House Canada, a division of
Random House of Canada Limited.

ISBN 978 0 7535 1322 4

Designed by Virgin Books Ltd

Printed and bound in Germany

Contents

Introduction

Ever since I wrote the original Gi Diet back in 2002, my mission has been to help as many people as possible lose weight and keep it off. It all began during my own personal struggle to lose weight. Though I had been working to raise awareness of heart disease and stroke as president of the Heart and Stroke Foundation of Ontario, and was earnestly promoting healthy lifestyle choices among Canadians to reduce their risk for those diseases, the sad truth was that I was overweight myself. In an effort to lose the extra pounds, I tried deprivation diet after starvation diet, weighed everything I put into my mouth, and calculated calories, points and carbs. But nothing I tried worked; I could never manage to lose more than a few pounds. It was so frustrating and demoralizing that if I hadn't felt duty-bound to 'walk the talk' as the chief representative of the Heart and Stroke Foundation of Ontario, I may well have given up. But I knew how dangerous my habits were to my health, and I doggedly persevered.

When eventually I found a diet based on the principles of the glycemic index, or Gi, which measures the speed at which your body breaks down carbohydrates and converts them to glucose, the vehicle your body uses for energy, I miraculously lost the extra weight that had been plaguing me for so long. I realised that, while I'd been blaming myself and my lack of willpower, the real reason I hadn't been able to slim down was that I didn't have the right information. I felt compelled to help other people who were trying to lose weight.

I persuaded my friends and associates to try the diet as well. But by the end of twelve months, 95 per cent of them had dropped out. I was so disappointed; I wanted to know why the diet hadn't worked for them. They gave two reasons: (1) The diet was too complicated to follow, requiring them to count grams and calculate formulas and ratios; and (2) they were always hungry. I felt that if I could solve these two fundamental problems, I could help people lose weight and improve their health. The result was The Gi Diet, a nutritionally ideal way to eat that emphasises fruits and vegetables, whole grains, low-fat dairy products, lean protein and the 'best' fats. As you can see, the Gi Diet doesn't eliminate any food groups. Its easy-to-follow colour-coded system means you will never have to count calories or points, or weigh and measure food. It will keep you feeling satisfied and energetic as you slim down to your ideal weight.

Since publication of The Gi Diet, I've received tens of thousands of letters from readers thrilled with their weight loss. The diet proved so successful that word quickly spread and, to date, over two million copies have been sold in seventeen languages in twenty-two countries.

Desperation is a major theme in the letters I receive. Many of them sound something like this: 'I have struggled with my weight all my life and I've tried everything – Weight Watchers, Jenny Craig, Atkins etc. – and despite some short-term success, I'm always back where I started, or worse. Help!' Those who have an above-average amount of weight to lose find they have an even harder battle. Their problem is not only the amount of weight they want to lose, but also their fear of failure and their low self-esteem. Virtually all have struggled with being overweight or obese for most of their lives, frequently since childhood. For them, food is a fickle friend who gives them a short-term feeling of wellbeing and comfort, but undermines their health, appearance and self-confidence.

Given the additional challenges facing people with an above-average amount of weight to lose, I decided to run a special programme through my website. I asked those who had a body mass index (BMI) of 33 or over – in other words, the clinically obese – to participate in an 'e-Clinic'. For thirteen weeks, I would send them a weekly e-mail introducing them to the basics of the Gi Diet, teaching them how to shop, cook and eat out, coaching them through the hurdles and helping them develop strategies for dealing with cravings and the emotional reasons we eat. In return, participants would send me their measurements and a diary each week. At the end of the thirteen weeks – enough time for people to get a good grasp of the diet and feel committed to the programme – we would switch to a monthly e-mail and diary.

Though hundreds of people applied, I could choose only forty to participate in the clinic. Remarkably, over 80 per cent of these 'hard cases' stuck with it until the end, and those who dropped out had to for the most part because of unrelated health problems. By the end of the first thirteen weeks, the average weight loss was an almost two stone! And I had received a wealth of feedback that I know will be tremendously helpful to others trying to achieve their weight-loss goals.

It's all here in The Gi Diet Clinic. Part One explains the principles behind the Gi Diet and how it works. Part Two is the thirteen-week guide that will get you started and coach you through all the challenges and pitfalls of following a new way of eating. Each week's guide includes a meal plan, grocery list and excerpts from e-Clinic participants' diaries. You will find these comments, stories, stumbling blocks and achievements relevant to your own experiences.

At the end of the thirteen weeks, you will be invited to sign on for a further nine monthly e-mail letters that will provide the latest news on green-light products as well as recipes and tips. You will also be invited to submit your own monthly diary and measurements. The e-mail letters will also provide valuable updates on the experiences and progress of other e-Clinic members.

So if you have tried diet after diet with no success, then this is the proven programme for you. Whether you have two stone or ten stone (or more) to lose, The Gi Diet Clinic will lead you every step of the way towards losing those extra pounds and inches, and, as importantly, keeping them off.

1

The Truth about Carbs, Fats and Protein

It's just about impossible to live in this country and not know that we are in the midst of an 'obesity epidemic'. If you watch television, listen to the radio, read the newspaper or simply notice the magazine headlines at the supermarket checkout, you can't help but be aware that over half of British people are overweight and that our obesity rate has doubled over the past twenty years. Everyone seems to have an explanation for our collective weight crisis: some hold the fast-food industry responsible; others blame our sedentary lifestyle; some maintain we are eating too much fat; others say we are eating too many carbohydrates. So what's the truth?

Well, all of these reasons are part of the answer. But if you reduce the problem to its physiological cause, it's actually quite simple: we're consuming more calories than we're expending, and the resulting surplus is stored around our waists, hips and thighs as fat. There's no mystery here. But to understand why we are consuming more calories, we need to get back to basics and look at the three fundamental elements of our diet: carbohydrates, fats and protein. We need to understand the role these components play in the digestive system and how they work together – whether we're in the process of getting fat or thin.

We'll start with carbohydrates, since the popularity of low-carbohydrate diets like the Atkins programme has made them a hot topic and given them a bad rap. Carbohydrates have been so much in the news over the past few years that a new word – 'carbs' – has entered the language. Though they've been blamed for all our weight problems, their role in weight control has really been misunderstood.

Carbohydrates

Carbohydrates are a necessary part of a healthy diet. They are rich in fibre, vitamins and minerals, including antioxidants, which we now know play an important role in the prevention of heart disease and cancer. Carbohydrates are also the primary source of energy for our bodies. They are found in grains, vegetables, fruits, legumes (beans) and dairy products.

Here is how carbs work: when you eat an orange or a bagel, your body digests the carbohydrates in the food and turns them into glucose, which provides you with energy. The glucose dissolves in your bloodstream and then travels to the parts of your body that use energy, such as your muscles and brain. So carbs are critical to everyone's health. When managing weight, however, it is important to realise that not all carbs are created equal.

Some carbohydrates break down into glucose in the digestive system at a slow and steady rate, gradually releasing their nutrients and keeping us feeling full and satisfied. Others break down rapidly, spiking our glucose levels and then disappearing quickly, leaving us feeling hungry again. For example, cornflakes and old-fashioned, large-flake oatmeal are both carbohydrates, but we all know the difference between eating a bowl of oatmeal for breakfast and eating a bowl of cornflakes. The oatmeal stays with you – it 'sticks to your ribs,' as my mother used to say – whereas your stomach starts rumbling an hour after eating the cornflakes, pushing you towards your next snack or meal. Throughout the course of a day, if you are eating carbs that break down rapidly, like cornflakes, as opposed to those that break down slowly, you will be eating more and, as a result, will begin to put on weight. If, however, you start eating carbs that break down slowly, like old-fashioned oatmeal, you will eat less and begin to lose weight. Selecting the right type of carb is key to achieving your optimum energy and weight. But how do you know which carbohydrate is the right type and which isn't?

Well, the first clue is the amount of processing that the food has undergone. The more a food is processed beyond its natural, fibrous state, the less processing your body has to do to digest it. The quicker you digest the food, the sooner you feel hungry again. This helps explain why the number of British adults who are overweight has surged over the last fifty years. A hundred years ago, most of the food people ate came straight from the farm to the dinner table. Lack of refrigeration and scant knowledge of food chemistry meant that most food remained in its original state. However, advances in science, along with the migration of many women out of the kitchen and into the workforce, led to a revolution in prepared foods geared to speed and simplicity of preparation. The giant food companies – Kraft, Kellogg's, Del Monte, Nestlé etc. – were born. We happily began spending more money for the convenience of prepared, processed, packaged, canned, frozen and bottled food. The 'ready meal' era had begun.

It was during this period that the miller's traditional wind and water mills were replaced with high-speed steel rolling mills, which stripped away most of the key nutrients, including the bran, fibre and wheat germ (which could spoil), to produce a talcum-like powder: today's white flour! This fine white flour is the basic ingredient for most of our breads and cereals, as well as for baked goods and snacks such as cookies, muffins, crackers and pretzels. Walk through any supermarket and you will be surrounded by towering stacks of these flour-based processed products. And we're eating more and more of these foods; over the past three decades, our consumption of grain has increased by 50 per cent. Our bodies are paying the price for this radical change in eating habits.

The second clue in determining whether a carbohydrate is the right type is the amount of fibre it contains. Fibre, in simple terms, provides low-calorie filler. It does double duty, in fact: it literally fills up your stomach, so you feel satiated; and your body takes much longer to break it down, so it stays with you longer and slows the digestive process. There are two forms of fibre: soluble and insoluble. Soluble fibre is found in carbs such as oatmeal, beans, barley and citrus fruits, and has been shown to lower blood cholesterol levels. Insoluble fibre is important for normal bowel function and is typically found in wholemeal breads and cereals, and most vegetables.

There are two other important components that inhibit the rapid breakdown of food in our digestive system, and they are fats and protein. Let's look at fats first.

Fats

Fat, like fibre, acts as a brake in the digestive process. When combined with other foods, fat becomes a barrier to digestive juices. It also signals the brain that you are satisfied and do not require more food. Does this mean that we should eat all the fat we want? Definitely not!

Though fat is essential for a nutritious diet, containing various key elements that are crucial to the digestive process, cell development and overall health, it also contains twice the number of calories per gram as carbohydrates and protein. If you decide to 'just add peanut butter' to your otherwise disciplined regime, it doesn't take much of it – two tablespoons – to spike your total calorie count. As well, once you eat fat, your body is a genius at hanging on to it and refusing to let it go. This is because fat is how the body stores reserve supplies of energy, usually around the waist, hips and thighs. Fat is money in the bank as far as the body is concerned – a rainy-day investment for when you have to call up extra energy. This clever system originally helped our ancestors survive during periods of famine. The problem today is that we don't live with cycles of feast and famine – it's more like feast, and then feast again! But the body's eagerness for fat continues, along with its reluctance to give it up.

This is why losing weight is so difficult: your body does everything it can to persuade you to eat more fat. How? Through fat's capacity to make things taste good. So it's not just you who thinks that juicy steaks, chocolate cake and rich ice cream taste better than a bean sprout. That's the fat content of cake and steak talking.

Sorry to say, there's no getting around it: if you want to lose weight, you have to watch your fat consumption. In addition, you need to be concerned about the type of fats you eat; many fats are harmful to your health. There are four types of fat: the best, the good, the bad and the really ugly. The 'really ugly' fats are potentially the most dangerous, and they lurk in many of our most popular snack foods. They are vegetable oils that have been heat-treated to make them thicken – the trans fats you've been hearing so much about in the media lately. They raise the amount of LDL, or bad, cholesterol in our bodies while lowering the amount of HDL, or good, cholesterol, which protects us from heart disease. As a result, they boost our cholesterol levels, which thickens our arteries and causes heart attack and stroke. So avoid using trans fats, such as vegetable shortening and hard margarine, and avoid packaged snack foods, baked goods, crackers and cereals that contain them. (You can spot them by checking labels for 'hydrogenated' or 'partially hydrogenated' oils.)

The 'bad' fats are called saturated fats and almost always come from animal sources. Butter, cheese and meat are all high in saturated fats. There are a couple of others you should be aware of too: coconut oil and palm oil are two vegetable oils that are saturated and, because they are cheap, they are used in many snack foods, especially cookies. Saturated fats, such as butter or cheese, are solid at room temperature. They elevate your risk of heart disease and Alzheimer's. The evidence is also growing that many cancers, including colon, prostate and breast cancer, are associated with diets high in saturated fats.

The 'good' fats are the polyunsaturated ones, and they are cholesterol free. Most vegetable oils, such as corn and sunflower, fall into this category. What you really should be eating, however, are the 'best' fats, the monounsaturated fats, which actually promote good health. These are the fats found in olives, almonds, and vegetable and olive oils. Monounsaturated fats have a beneficial effect on cholesterol and are good for your heart. This is one reason the incidence of heart disease is low in Mediterranean countries, where olive oil is a staple. Although fancy olive oil is expensive, you can enjoy the same health benefits from less costly supermarket brands.

Another highly beneficial oil that falls into the 'best' category is omega-3, a fatty acid found in deep-sea fish, such as salmon, mackerel, albacore tuna and herring, as well as in lake trout, walnuts, and flaxseed oil. Some brands of eggs (e.g. Columbus) also contain omega-3, which can help lower cholesterol and protect cardiovascular health.

So the 'best' and 'good' fats are an important part of a healthy diet and also help slow digestion. Still, they're fat and they pack a lot of calories. We have to be careful, then, to limit our intake of polyunsaturated fats when trying to lose weight.

Since protein also acts as a brake in the digestive process, let's look at it in more detail.

Protein

Protein is an absolutely essential part of your diet. In fact, you are already half protein: 50 per cent of your dry body weight is made up of muscles, organs, skin and hair, all forms of protein. We need this element to build and repair body tissues, and it figures in nearly all metabolic reactions. Protein is also a critical brain food, providing amino acids for the neurotransmitters that relay messages to the brain. This is why it's not a good idea to skip breakfast on the morning of a big meeting or exam. The 'brain fog' people experience on some diets is likely to be the result of diminished protein. Protein is literally food for thought.

The main sources of dietary protein come from animals: meat, seafood, dairy and eggs. Vegetable sources include beans and soya-based products such as tofu. Unfortunately, protein sources such as red meat and full-fat dairy products are also high in 'bad', or saturated, fats, which are harmful to your health. It is important that we get our protein from sources that are low in saturated fats, such as lean meats, skinless poultry, seafood, low-fat dairy products, egg whites, and tofu and other soya products.

One exceptional source of protein is the humble bean. Beans are a perfect food, really: they're high in protein and fibre, and low in saturated fat. No wonder so many of the world's cuisines have found myriad wonderful ways to cook beans. We need to become more bean savvy. Nuts are another excellent source of protein and are relatively low in fat – as long as you don't eat a whole bowlful.

Protein is much more effective than carbohydrates or fat at satisfying hunger. It will make you feel fuller longer, which is why you should try to incorporate some protein into every meal and snack. This will help keep you on the ball and feeling satisfied.

Now that we know how carbohydrates, fats and protein work in our digestive system, let's use the science to discover how to take off the extra pounds.

TO SUM UP

1. Eat carbohydrates that have not been highly processed and that do not contain highly processed ingredients.

2. Eat less fat overall and look for low-fat alternatives to your current food choices.

3. Eat only monounsaturated and polyunsaturated fats.

4. Include some protein in all your meals and snacks.

5. Eat low-fat protein only, preferably from both animal and vegetable sources.

2

The Secret to Easy, Permanent Weight Loss

The 'Gi' in Gi Diet stands for glycemic index, which is the basis of this diet – and the only scientific phrase you'll need to know. The glycemic index is the secret to reducing calories and losing weight without going hungry. It measures the speed at which carbohydrates break down in our digestive system and turn into glucose, the body's main source of energy or fuel.

The glycemic index was developed by Dr David Jenkins, a professor of nutritional sciences at the University of Toronto, when he was researching the impact of different carbohydrates on the blood sugar, or glucose, level of diabetics. He found that certain carbohydrates broke down quickly and flooded the bloodstream with sugar, but others broke down more slowly, only marginally increasing blood-sugar levels. The faster a food breaks down, the higher its rating on the glycemic index, which sets sugar at 100 and scores all other foods against that number. These findings were important to diabetics, who could then use the index to identify low-Gi, slow-release foods that would help control their blood-sugar levels. Here are some examples of the Gi ratings of a range of popular foods:

Examples of Gi ratings

High Gi	Low Gi
Baguette 95	Orange 44
Cornflakes 84	All-Bran 43
Rice cake 82	Oatmeal 42
Doughnut 76	Spaghetti 41
Bagel 72	Apple 38
Cereal bar 72	Beans 31
Biscuit 69	Plain yoghurt 25

What do these Gi ratings have to do with the numbers on your bathroom scale? Well, it turns out that low-Gi, slow-release foods have a significant impact on our ability to lose weight. As I have explained, when we eat the wrong type of carb, a high-Gi food, the body quickly digests it and releases a flood of sugar (glucose) into the bloodstream. This gives us a short-term high, but the sugar is just as quickly absorbed by the body, leaving us with a post-sugar slump. We feel lethargic and start looking for our next sugar fix. A fast-food lunch of a double cheeseburger, fries and a Coke delivers a short-term burst of energy, but by mid-afternoon we start feeling tired, sluggish and hungry. That's when we reach for 'just one' brownie or bag of potato chips. These high-Gi foods deliver the rush we want and then let us down again. The roller-coaster ride is a hard cycle to break. But a high-Gi diet will make you feel hungry more often, so you end up eating more and gaining more weight.

Let's look at the other end of the Gi index. Low-Gi foods, such as fruits, vegetables, whole grains, pasta, beans and low-fat dairy products, take longer to digest, deliver a steady supply of sugar to our bloodstream and leave us feeling fuller for a longer time. Consequently, we eat less. It also helps that these foods are lower in calories. As a result, we consume less food and fewer calories, without going hungry or feeling unsatisfied.

The key player in this process of energy storage and retrieval is insulin, a hormone secreted by the pancreas. Insulin does two things very well. First, it regulates the amount of sugar (glucose) in our bloodstream, removing the excess and storing it as glycogen for immediate use by our muscles, or putting it into storage as fat. Second, insulin acts as a security guard at the fat gates, reluctantly giving up its reserves. This evolutionary feature is a throwback to the days when our ancestors were hunter-gatherers, habitually experiencing times of feast or famine. When food was in abundance, the body stored its surplus as fat to tide it over the inevitable days of famine.

A few years ago, I was on vacation in a remote part of central Mexico, visiting the Copper Canyon, which, incredibly, is larger and deeper than the Grand Canyon in Arizona. A tribe of Tarahumara Indians still resides there. Until recently, these indigenous peoples typically put on two stone during the summer and fall, when the crops, particularly corn, were plentiful. Then, over the course of the winter, when food became scarce, they lost these two stone. Insulin was the champion in this process, both helping to accumulate fat and then guarding its depletion.

Of course, food is now readily available to us at the nearest twenty-four-hour supermarket. But our bodies still function very much as they did in the earliest days. When we eat a high-Gi food, our pancreas releases insulin to reduce the glucose level in our blood, which, if left unchecked, would lead to hyperglycaemia. If we aren't using all that energy at the moment, the glucose is stored as fat. Soon we become hungry again. Our body can either draw on our reserves of fat and laboriously convert them back to sugar, or it can look for more food. Since giving up extra fat is the body's last choice – who knows when that supply might come in handy! – our body would rather send us to the fridge than work to convert fat back to sugar. This helped our survival back in the old days, but it gets in the way of weight loss now.

So our goal is to limit the amount of insulin in our system by avoiding high-Gi foods, which stimulate its production, and instead choosing low-Gi foods, which keep the supply of sugar in our bloodstream consistent. Slow-release, low- Gi carbohydrates help curb your appetite by leaving you feeling fuller for a longer period of time. When you combine them with lean protein and the best fats, which help slow the digestive process, you have the magic combination that will allow you to lose weight without going hungry.

Translated into real food, what does this mean? Well, for dinner you could have a grilled chicken breast, boiled new potatoes, a side salad of Cos lettuce and red pepper dressed with a bit of olive oil and lemon juice, and some asparagus if you feel like it. The trick is to stick with foods that have a low Gi, are low in fat and are low-ish in calories. This sounds – and is, in fact – quite complex. It might seem to you as though I'm breaking my promise of an easy weight-loss plan. But don't worry: I've done all the calculations, measurements and maths for you, and sorted the foods you like to eat into one of three categories based on the colours of the traffic light. On pages 191–204, you will find the Complete Gi Diet Food Guide, which has a list of foods in a red column, a list in a yellow column, and a list in a green column. Here's how the colour-coded categories work:

Red-light foods
The foods in the red column are to be avoided. They are high-Gi, higher-calorie foods that will make it impossible for you to lose weight.

Yellow-light foods
The foods in the yellow column are mid-range-Gi foods that should be treated with caution. They should be avoided when you are trying to lose weight, but once you've slimmed down to your ideal weight, you can begin to enjoy yellow-light foods from time to time.

Green-light foods
The green column lists foods that are low-Gi, low in fat and lower in calories. These are the foods that will allow you to lose weight. Don't expect them to be tasteless and boring! There are many delicious and satisfying choices that will make you feel as though you aren't even on a diet.

If you're a veteran of the low-carbohydrate craze, you'll be surprised to find potatoes and rice in the green-light column; but they are fine as long as they are the right type. Baked potatoes and French fries have a high Gi, while boiled new potatoes have a low Gi. The short-grain, glutinous rice served in Chinese and Thai restaurants is high-Gi, while long-grain, brown, basmati and wild rice are low-Gi. Pasta is also a green-light food – as long as it is cooked only until al dente (with some firmness to the bite). Any processing of food, including cooking, increases a food's Gi, since heat breaks down starch capsules and fibre, giving your digestive juices a head start. This is why you should never overcook vegetables; instead, steam them or boil them in a small amount of water just until they are tender. This way, they will retain their vitamins and other nutrients, and their Gi rating will remain low.

While eating green-light foods is really the core of the Gi Diet, there are a few more things you'll need to know to follow the programme. Let's discuss these in the next chapter.

TO SUM UP

1. Low-Gi foods take longer to digest, so you feel satiated longer.

2. The key to losing weight is to eat low-Gi, low-calorie foods – in other words, foods from the green-light column of the Complete Gi Diet Food Guide (see pages 191–204).

3

The Gi Diet Essentials

The Gi Diet consists of two phases. For those with a more serious weight problem, an additional Preliminary Phase has been added. The preliminary phase and phase 1 are the dramatic parts of the Gi Diet – the period when those extra unwanted pounds come off! During these stages, you'll focus on eating foods that are low- Gi and also low in fat and sugar – the foods in the green-light column of the Complete Gi Diet Food Guide on pages 191–204. Yes, this means a farewell to bagels and a fond adieu to Häagen-Dazs. But it doesn't mean you won't have a multitude of delicious foods to choose from. Once you've slimmed down to your ideal weight, you enter Phase II, the maintenance phase of the programme, which is the way you will eat for the rest of your life.

To decide whether you will be starting with the Preliminary Phase or Phase I, you will need to find out your Body Mass Index (BMI), which is a measurement of how much body fat you are carrying relative to your height.

Your BMI

While the BMI gives a relatively accurate measure of body fat, it applies only to people who are 20 to 65 years of age. It isn't valid for children, pregnant or nursing women, the elderly or heavily muscled athletes. For the rest of us, however, it is the only accepted international standard for weight.

You can calculate your BMI from the table on pages 18–19. Simply find your height in the horizontal row along the top of the table. Then run your finger down the column until it's in line with your weight in the vertical column on the left. The figure in the chart where your two measurements intersect is your BMI.

If your BMI falls between 19 and 24, your weight is within the acceptable norm and is considered healthy. Anything between 25 and 29 is considered overweight; if you're 30 or over, you are officially obese.

If your BMI is 32 or under I recommend you begin with Phase I of the programme. If it's over 32 then start with the Preliminary Phase.

The Preliminary Phase and Phase I

Now you know if you'll be starting with the Preliminary Phase or Phase I, it's time to get into the details: what to eat, how much and how often.

What do I eat?

As you know, during the Preliminary Phase and Phase I, you will be sticking to the foods listed in the green-light column of the Complete Gi Diet Food Guide on pages 191–204.

How much do I eat?

Remember, this is not a starvation diet – far from it. Going hungry is simply not necessary for weight loss; in fact, it's something to be resolutely avoided! If you are hungry for a sustained period of time, your body will feel that it hasn't received enough fuel to meet its needs and will slow the rate at which it burns calories, making it even harder to lose those extra pounds. So never leave your digestive system with nothing to do. If your digestive system is busy processing food and steadily supplying energy to your brain, not only will your metabolism keep firing at a steady rate, but also you won't be looking for high-calorie snacks. This is why you can, for the most part, eat as much green-light food as you want on the Gi Diet.

In Phase I, you should be eating three meals and three snacks every day. And in the Preliminary Phase, you should be eating three meals and four snacks every day. The reason I recommend an extra snack in the Preliminary Phase is because someone with a larger body requires more calories just to keep functioning on a daily basis than someone who is lighter. This is also why I suggest larger serving sizes for some green-light foods in the Preliminary Phase than in Phase I. Although I generally do not restrict quantities of green-light foods – within reason (five heads of cabbage is a bit extreme) – there are a few exceptions, which I outline below. (Except where indicated, a serving size is per meal, not per day.)

Green-light Servings

Green-Light Food	Preliminary Phase (BMI of 33 or more)	Phase I (BMI of 32 or less)
Crispbreads (with high fibre)	3	2
Green-light breads (which have at least 2.5–3g of fibre per slice)	2 slices per day	1 slice per day
Green-light cereals	60g (2oz)	50g (1 ⅔oz)
Green-light nuts	12 to 15	8 to 10
Margarine (soft, non-hydrogenated, light)	3tsp	2tsp
Meat, fish, poultry	180g (6oz)	120g (4oz) (about the size of a pack of cards)
Olive/vegetable oil	1 ½tsp	1tsp
Olives	6 to 8	4 to 5
Pasta	55g (1 ¾oz)	40g (1 ½oz uncooked)
Potatoes (new, boiled)	4 to 5	2 to 3
Rice (basmati, brown, long-grain)	65g (2 ¼oz uncooked)	50g (1 ¾oz uncooked)

BMI TABLE

british stones	british lbs	us pounds	kilos	4'6" (137)	4'8" (142)	4'10" (147)	5'0" (152)	5'2" (157)	5'3" (160)	5'4" (163)	5'5" (165)	5'6" (168)	5'7" (170)	5'8" (173)	5'9" (175)	5'10" (178)	5'11" (180)	6'0" (183)	6'2" (188)	6'4" (193)	6'6" (198)	6'8" (203)
6	7	91	41	22.0	20.4	19.0	17.8	16.6	16.1	15.6	15.1	14.7	14.3	13.8	13.4	13.1	12.7	12.3	11.7	11.1	10.5	10.0
6	10	94	43	22.7	21.1	19.6	18.4	17.2	16.7	16.1	15.6	15.2	14.7	14.3	13.9	13.5	13.1	12.7	12.1	11.4	10.9	10.3
7	0	98	44	23.7	22.0	20.5	19.1	17.9	17.4	16.8	16.3	15.8	15.3	14.9	14.5	14.1	13.7	13.3	12.6	11.9	11.3	10.8
7	3	101	46	24.4	22.6	21.1	19.7	18.5	17.9	17.3	16.8	16.3	15.8	15.4	14.9	14.5	14.1	13.7	13.0	12.3	11.7	11.1
7	7	105	48	25.4	23.5	21.9	20.5	19.2	18.6	18.0	17.5	16.9	16.4	16.0	15.5	15.1	14.6	14.2	13.5	12.8	12.1	11.5
7	10	108	49	26.1	24.2	22.6	21.1	19.8	19.1	18.5	18.0	17.4	16.9	16.4	15.9	15.5	15.1	14.6	13.9	13.1	12.5	11.9
8	0	112	51	27.1	25.1	23.4	21.9	20.5	19.8	19.2	18.6	18.1	17.5	17.0	16.5	16.1	15.6	15.2	14.4	13.6	12.9	12.3
8	3	115	52	27.8	25.8	24.0	22.5	21.0	20.4	19.7	19.1	18.6	18.0	17.5	17.0	16.5	16.0	15.6	14.8	14.0	13.3	12.6
8	7	119	54	28.8	26.7	24.9	23.2	21.8	21.1	20.4	19.8	19.2	18.6	18.1	17.6	17.1	16.6	16.1	15.3	14.5	13.8	13.1
8	10	122	55		27.4	25.5	23.8	22.3	21.6	20.9	20.3	19.7	19.1	18.5	18.0	17.5	17.0	16.5	15.7	14.9	14.1	13.4
9	3	129	59		28.9	27.0	25.2	23.6	22.9	22.1	21.5	21.0	20.2	19.6	19.0	18.5	18.0	17.5	16.6	15.7	14.9	14.2
9	7	133	60			27.8	26.0	24.3	23.6	22.8	22.1	21.5	20.8	20.2	19.6	19.1	18.5	18.0	17.1	16.2	15.4	14.6
9	10	136	62			28.4	26.6	24.9	24.1	23.3	22.6	22.0	21.3	20.7	20.1	19.5	19.0	18.4	17.5	16.6	15.7	14.9
10	0	140	64			29.3	27.3	25.6	24.8	24.0	23.3	22.6	21.9	21.3	20.7	20.1	19.5	19.0	18.0	17.0	16.2	15.4
10	3	143	65				27.9	26.2	25.3	24.5	23.8	23.1	22.4	21.7	21.1	20.5	19.9	19.4	18.4	17.4	16.5	15.7
10	7	147	67				28.7	26.9	26.0	25.2	24.5	23.7	23.0	22.4	21.7	21.1	20.5	19.9	18.9	17.9	17.0	16.1
10	10	150	68					27.4	26.6	25.7	25.0	24.2	23.5	22.8	22.2	21.5	20.9	20.3	19.3	18.3	17.3	16.5
11	0	154	70					28.2	27.3	26.4	25.6	24.9	24.1	23.4	22.7	22.1	21.5	20.9	19.8	18.7	17.8	16.9
11	3	157	71					28.7	27.8	26.9	26.1	25.3	24.6	23.9	23.2	22.5	21.9	21.3	20.2	19.1	18.1	17.2
11	7	161	73						28.5	27.6	26.8	26.0	25.2	24.5	23.8	23.1	22.5	21.8	20.7	19.6	18.6	17.7
11	10	164	74						29.1	28.2	27.3	26.5	25.7	24.9	24.2	23.5	22.9	22.2	21.1	20.0	19.0	18.0
12	0	168	76							28.8	28.0	27.1	26.3	25.5	24.8	24.1	23.4	22.8	21.6	20.4	19.4	18.5
12	3	171	78								28.5	27.6	26.8	26.0	25.3	24.5	23.8	23.2	22.0	20.8	19.8	18.8
12	7	175	79								29.1	28.2	27.4	26.6	25.8	25.1	24.4	23.7	22.5	21.3	20.2	19.2

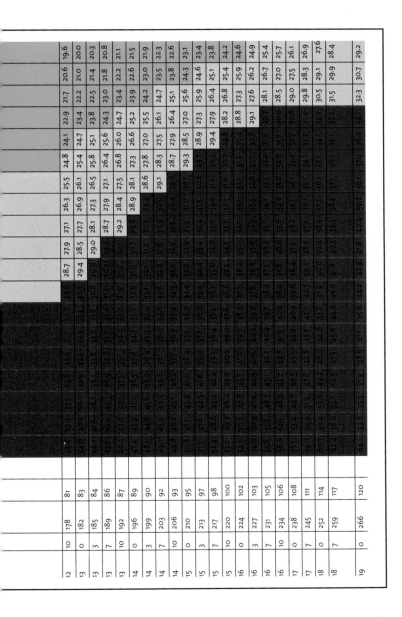

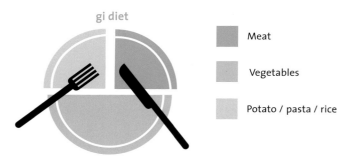

gi diet

- Meat
- Vegetables
- Potato / pasta / rice

Each meal and snack should contain, if possible, a combination of green-light protein, carbohydrates – especially vegetables and fruit – and fats. An easy way to visualise portion size is to divide your plate into three sections (see illustration above). Half the plate should be filled with vegetables; one-quarter should contain protein, such as lean meat, poultry, seafood, eggs, tofu or legumes; and the last quarter should contain a green-light serving of rice, pasta or potatoes.

When do I eat?

Try to eat regularly throughout the day. If you skimp on breakfast and lunch, you will probably be starving by dinner and end up piling on the food. Have one snack mid-morning, another mid-afternoon and the last before bed. In the Preliminary Phase, the fourth snack can be eaten later in the afternoon if you usually have a late dinner, or during the evening if you generally have an early dinner. It's really up to you – have the extra snack at the time of day when you feel you most need it. The idea is to keep your digestive system happily busy so you won't start craving those red-light snacks.

Meal basics

Because the green-light way of eating is most likely new to you, you're probably wondering what to eat instead of that bagel with cream cheese for breakfast, that hamburger for lunch, and those tortilla chips and salsa for a snack. On the following pages, I'll go over your various green-light options for each of the main meals and snacks of your daily Gi programme. Let's start with breakfast.

Breakfast

I know you've been told that breakfast is the most important meal of the day, and it's actually true. It's the first thing you eat after your night-long 'fast' of twelve hours or more, and it launches you into your workday. Eating a healthy breakfast will help you avoid the need to grab a coffee and Danish as soon as you hit the office, and will make you feel satisfied and energetic. Eating breakfast every day doesn't mean you have to set the alarm any earlier. If you have time to read the paper or feed the cat, you have time to prepare and eat a green-light breakfast.

The following chart lists typical breakfast foods in the colour-coded categories. To ensure you have a balanced breakfast, include some green-light carbohydrates, protein and fat. For a complete list of foods, see the Complete Gi Diet Food Guide on pages 191–204.

PROTEIN	Red	Yellow	Green
Meat, poultry and eggs	Regular bacon Sausages Whole regular eggs	Turkey bacon Whole omega-3 eggs	Back bacon Lean deli ham Egg whites
Dairy	Cheese Cottage cheese (regular) Cream Milk (whole) Sour cream Yoghurt (regular)	Cream cheese (light) Milk (semi-skimmed) Sour cream (light) Yoghurt (low-fat with sugar)	Buttermilk Cheese (fat-free) Cottage cheese (low-fat or fat-free) Fruit yoghurt (non-fat with sugar substitute) Milk (skimmed) Soya milk (plain, low-fat)
CARBOHYDRATES			
Cereals	All cold cereals except those listed as amber- or green-light Granola Muesli (commercial)	Shredded wheat	All-Bran Oat Bran Porridge (traditional large-flake e.g. Jordan's)
Breads/grains	Bagels Baguettes Biscuits Doughnuts Muffins Pancakes Waffles White bread	Crispbreads (with fibre) Wholemeal breads*	100% stone-ground wholemeal bread* Crispbreads (with fibre, e.g. Ryvita High Fibre) Green-light muffins (see pages 181–3) Wholemeal high-fibre breads (2.5–3g fibre per slice)*
Fruits	Apple puree (containing sugar) Tinned fruit in syrup Melons Most dried fruit	Apricots (fresh and dried)** Bananas Dried cranberries** Fruit cocktail in juice Kiwi Mango Papaya Pineapple	Apples Berries Cherries Grapefruit Grapes Oranges Peaches Plums
Juices	Fruit drinks Prune Sweetened juices Watermelon	Apple (unsweetened) Grapefruit (unsweetened) Orange (unsweetened) Pear (unsweetened)	Eat the fruit rather than drink its juice
Vegetables	Chips Hash browns		Most vegetables
FATS			
Fats	Butter Hard margarine Peanut butter (regular and light) Tropical oils Vegetable shortening	Most nuts 100% peanut butter Soft margarine (non-hydrogenated) Vegetable oils	Almonds* Hazelnuts* Olive oil* Soft margarine (non-hydrogenated, light)*

* Limit serving size (see page 17).
** For baking, it is OK to use a modest amount of dried apricots or cranberries.

Let's take a closer look at some of the usual breakfast choices.

Coffee and tea

OK, this is the toughest one. The trouble with coffee is caffeine. It's not a health problem in itself, but it does stimulate the production of insulin. That's part of the 'buzz' we get from coffee. But insulin reduces blood-sugar levels, which then increases your appetite. Have you ever ordered a Venti from Starbucks and then felt positively shaky an hour later? That's your blood sugar hitting bottom. You cure it by eating a bagel – which isn't helpful when you're trying to lose weight. So in Phase I, try to cut out caffeine altogether. As unpleasant as it may be, caffeine withdrawal will end in a day or two. Cut down gradually: go from a medium coffee to a small; then try a half-caffeinated–half-decaf blend. Then limit yourself to decaffeinated coffee – some brands taste as good as the real thing.

Even better, switch to tea. It has only about one-third of the caffeine that coffee has, and black tea and green tea have health benefits as well: they're rich in antioxidants, and beneficial for heart health and reducing the risk of dementia. Green tea is also considered an anti-carcinogen. (My ninety-seven-year-old mother and her tea-drinking cronies are living proof!) Herbal teas, such as peppermint, chamomile and other blends, are fine, too, as long as they contain no caffeine.

If going without coffee altogether is going to be a real problem, then go ahead, have one cup a day – but not a double espresso. If you take milk and sugar, make it skimmed milk and a sweetener such as Splenda.

Cereals

Another toughie. Most cold cereals contain hidden or not-so-hidden sugars, and are therefore red-light. Green-light cereals are high in fibre; they have at least 10g per serving. All right, they're not a lot of fun by themselves, but you can liven them up with fresh, canned or frozen fruits, a few nuts and some fruit yoghurt (fat-free, with sugar substitute).

My personal favourite cereal is good old-fashioned porridge oats – not the instant type that comes in packets but the large-flake, slow-cooking kind. (They're starting to serve it in the smartest hotels now.) Large-flake porridge oats are not only low-Gi, but also low-calorie and have been shown to lower cholesterol. Yes, you have to cook it, but it takes only about three minutes or so in the microwave, and not much longer for one portion on top of the cooker. Dress it up with yoghurt, sliced almonds, berries or unsweetened apple sauce. It's also just fine with nothing but milk on it. I probably receive more e-mails about people's delight at rediscovering oatmeal than about any other food or meal. Give it a try.

Toast

Go ahead, but have no more than one slice per meal. Make sure your bread has at least 2.5–3g of fibre per slice. (Note: Some bread labels quote a two-slice serving, which should equal 5–6g per serving.) The best choice is 100% stone-ground wholemeal bread, which has a coarser grind and therefore a lower Gi. White bread, cracked wheat or anything else made with white flour is red-light.

Butter and jams

Butter is out. It's very high in saturated fat, and despite the protestations of the dairy industry, it's not good for your health or waistline. Yes, it does make things taste good – that's what fat does best. But you can still enjoy any one of a variety of light non-hydrogenated soft margarines, if you use only a teaspoon or so.

When buying fruit spreads, look for the 'extra fruit'/'no sugar added' varieties. Fruit, not sugar, should be the first ingredient listed. These varieties taste great and don't have the calories of the usual commercial jams.

Dairy

Low-fat dairy products are an ideal green-light choice and an excellent source of protein. I have a glass of skimmed milk every morning. I admit that skimmed probably won't taste great at first, but try weaning yourself off full-fat by switching to semi-skimmed before moving on to skimmed. Full-fat will then taste like cream!

Fat-free yoghurt with sugar substitute instead of sugar is ideal for break-fast, dessert or a snack, either by itself or added to fruits or cereals. Low-fat cottage cheese is also a top-rated green-light source of protein. Or you can make a low-fat soft cheese spread by letting yoghurt drain in cheesecloth overnight in the refrigerator.

Regular full-fat dairy products, including full-fat milk and cream, cheese and butter, are loaded with saturated fat and should be avoided completely.

Eggs

As whole eggs are a yellow-light food, try to use egg whites where possible. (If you're eating a hotel breakfast, in most cases the kitchen is happy to make omelettes with egg whites only.) Otherwise, use omega-3 whole eggs such as Columbus, but limit the number to seven per week. (Unless you have a medi-cal cholesterol problem, you can eat as many as you wish in Phase II.)

Bacon

Bacon is red-light because of its high saturated-fat content. However, there are tasty green-light alternatives – such as back bacon, turkey bacon and lean ham – that make great BLTs!

Lunch

Lunch is usually the most problematic meal for my readers because they tend to eat it outside the home and in a hurry. Bringing your lunch to work is the easiest way to ensure you eat green-light. And there are other advantages to taking a packed lunch besides avoiding the temptation of a red-light lunch: it's cheaper, and it gives you downtime at your desk to read or catch up on paperwork. Here are the ground rules for making that lunchbox a green-light one. For a complete list of foods, see the Complete Gi Diet Food Guide on Pages 191–204.

PROTEIN	Red	Yellow	Green
Meat, poultry fish, eggs and soy	Beef burgers Beef mince (more than 10% fat) Hot dogs Paté Processed meats Regular bacon Sausages Whole regular eggs	Beef mince (lean) Lamb (lean cuts) Pork (lean cuts) Tofu Turkey bacon Whole omega-3 eggs	All fish and seafood, fresh or frozen (not battered or breaded) or canned in water Beef (lean cuts) Beef mince (extra-lean) Chicken breast (skinless) Egg whites Tofu (low-fat) Turkey breast (skinless) Veal
CARBOHYDRATES			
Breads/grains	Bagels Baguettes Beef burger or hot dog buns Biscuits Cake Crispbreads Croissants Croutons Doughnuts Muffins Noodles Pancakes Pasta filled with cheese or meat Pizza Rice (short-grain, white, instant) Tortillas Waffles	Crispbreads (with fibre) Pitta (wholemeal) Wholemeal breads*	100% stone-ground wholemeal bread* Crispbreads (high-fibre, e.g. Ryvita High Fibre) Pasta (fettuccine, linguine, macaroni, penne, spaghetti) Quinoa Rice (basmati, wild, brown, long-grain) Wholemeal high-fibre breads (2.5–3g fibre per slice)*

Fruits and vegetables	Broad beans Chips Melons Most dried fruit Parsnips Potatoes (mashed or baked) Swede Turnip	Apricots Artichokes Bananas Beetroot Kiwi Mango Papaya Pineapple Potatoes (boiled) Squash Sweet corn Sweet potatoes	Apples Asparagus Aubergine Avocado* Beans (green/runner) Blackberries Broccoli Brussels sprouts Cabbage Carrots Cauliflower Celery Cherries Chilli peppers Courgettes Cucumber Grapefruit Grapes Leeks Lemons Lettuce Mangetout Mushrooms Olives* Onions Oranges (all varieties) Peaches Pears Peas Peppers (green and red) Pickles Plums Potatoes (new, boiled) Radishes Raspberries Rocket Spinach Strawberries Tomatoes
FATS			
Fats	Butter Hard margarine Mayonnaise (regular) Peanut butter (regular and light) Salad dressings (regular) Tropical oils Vegetable shortening	Mayonnaise (light) Most nut 100% peanut butter Salad dressings (light) Soft margarine (non-hydrogenated)	Almonds* Mayonnaise (fat free) Olive oil* Salad dressings (low fat, low-sugar) Soft margarine (non-hydrogenated, light)*
SOUPS			
Soups	All cream-based soups Tinned black bean Tinned green pea Tinned puréed vegetable Tinned split pea	Tinned chicken noodle Tinned lentil Tinned tomato	Chunky bean and vegetable soups (e.g. Baxter's Healthy Choice)

* Limit serving size (see page 17).

Sandwiches

Sandwiches are a lunchtime staple, and it's no wonder: they're portable, easy to make and offer endless variety. They can also be a dietary disaster, but if you follow the suggestions below, you can keep your sandwiches green-light:

1. Always use 100% stone-ground wholemeal or high-fibre whole-grain bread (2.5–3g of fibre per slice).

2. Sandwiches should be served open-faced. Either pack components separately and assemble just before eating or make your sandwich with a 'lettuce lining' that helps keep the bread from getting soggy.

3. Include at least three vegetables, such as lettuce, tomato, red or green pepper, cucumber, sprouts or onion.

4. Instead of spreading the bread with butter or margarine, use mustard or hummus.

5. Add up to 120g (4oz) of cooked lean meat or fish: roast beef, turkey, shrimp or salmon.

6. If you make tuna or chicken salad, use low-fat mayonnaise or low-fat salad dressing and celery.

7. Mix canned salmon with malt vinegar or fresh lemon.

Salads

Preparing salads may seem more labour intensive than making sandwiches, but it doesn't have to be. Invest in a variety of reusable plastic containers so you can bring individual-sized salads to work. Keep a supply of green-light vinaigrette on hand, and wash greens ahead of time and store in paper towels in plastic bags. You'll find that salads are a creative way to use up leftovers with a minimum of fuss.

Dinner

Dinner is traditionally the main meal of the day, and the one where we may have a tendency to overeat. We usually have more time for eating at the end of the day, and we generally feel fatigued as well, which encourages us to consume more. But since we will probably be spending the evening relaxing before going to bed rather than being active, it is important that we don't overdo it. For a complete list of foods, see the Complete Gi Diet Food Guide on Pages 191–204.

PROTEIN	Red	Yellow	Green
Meat, poultry fish and eggs	Beef burgers Beef mince (more than 10% fat) Breaded fish and seafood Fish tinned in oil Hot dogs Processed meats Sausages Sushi Whole regular eggs	Beef mince (lean) Lamb (lean cuts) Pork (lean cuts) Whole omega-3 eggs	All fish and seafood, fresh or frozen (not battered, breaded or tinned in oil) Beef (lean cuts) Beef mince (extra-lean) Chicken breast (skinless) Egg whites Lean deli ham Turkey breast (skinless) Veal
Dairy	Cheese Cottage cheese (regular) Milk (whole) Soured cream Yoghurt (regular)	Cheese (low-fat) Milk (semi-skimmed) Soured cream (light) Yoghurt (low-fat)	Cheese (fat free) Cottage cheese (fat free) Fruit yoghurt (non-fat with sugar substitute) Soya milk (plain, low fat)
CARBOHYDRATES			
Breads/grains	Bagels Baguettes Biscuits Cake Croissants Doughnuts Muffins Noodles Pasta filled with cheese or meat Pizza Rice (short-grain, white, instant) Tortillas	Pitta (wholemeal) Wholemeal breads*	100% stone-ground wholemeal bread* Pasta (fettuccine, linguine, macaroni, penne, spaghetti)* Quinoa Rice (basmati, wild, brown, long-grain) Wholemeal high-fibre breads (2.5–3g fibre per slice)*
Fruits and vegetables	Broad beans Chips Melons Most dried fruit Parsnips Potatoes (mashed or baked) Swede Turnip	Apricots Bananas Beetroot Kiwi Mango Papaya Pineapple Pomegranates Potatoes (boiled) Squash Sweet corn Sweet potatoes	Apples Asparagus Aubergine Avocado* Beans (green/runner) Blackberries Broccoli Brussels sprouts Cabbage Carrots Cauliflower Celery Cherries Chilli peppers Courgettes Cucumber Grapefruit Grapes Leeks Lemons Lettuce Mangetout Mushrooms **Continues on next page →**

Fruits and vegetables			Olives* Onions Oranges (all varieties) Peaches Pears Peas Peppers (green and red) Pickles Plums Potatoes (new, boiled) Radishes Raspberries Rocket Spinach Strawberries Tomatoes
FATS			
Fats	Butter Hard margarine Mayonnaise (regular) Peanut butter (regular and light) Salad dressings (regular) Tropical oils	Mayonnaise (light) Most nuts 100% peanut butter Salad dressings (light) Soft margarine (non-hydrogenated) Vegetable oils Walnuts	Almonds* Mayonnaise (fat free) Olive oil* Pistachios Salad dressings (low fat, low sugar) Soft margarine (non-hydrogenated, light)*
SOUPS			
Soups	All cream-based soups Tinned black bean Tinned green pea Tinned puréed vegetable Tinned split pea	Tinned chicken noodle Tinned lentil Tinned tomato	Chunky bean and vegetable soups (e.g. Baxter's Healthy Choice) Homemade soups with green-light ingredients

* Limit serving size (see Page 17).

The protein

No dinner is complete without protein. Whether it is in the form of meat, poultry, seafood, beans or tofu, it should cover no more than one-quarter of your plate. A serving size should be 120g (4oz) , which is roughly the size of the palm of your hand.

Red Meat

Though most red meat does contain saturated fat, there are ways to minimise it:

- Buy only low-fat meats such as topside of beef. For hamburgers or spaghetti sauces, buy extra-lean beef mince. Veal and pork tenderloin are low in fat, too. As for juicy steaks, well, they are juicy because of the fat in them, so they're not a good choice.

- Trim any visible fat from the meat. Even a quarter-inch of fat can double the total amount of fat in the meat.

- Broiling or grilling allows the excess fat from the meat to drain off. (Try one of those George Foreman–style fat-draining electric grills.)

- For stovetop cooking, use a non-stick pan with a little vegetable-oil spray rather than oil. The spray goes further.

Poultry

Skinless chicken and turkey breast are excellent green-light choices. In the yellow-light category are skinless thighs, wings and legs, which are higher in fat.

Seafood

This is always a good green-light choice. Although certain cold-water fish, such as salmon and cod, have a relatively high oil content, this oil is omega-3 and is beneficial to your heart health. Shrimp and squid are fine, too, as long as they aren't breaded or battered. Fish and chips, alas, are out.

Beans (legumes)

If you don't think you're into beans, it's time to re-evaluate! Beans are such an excellent source of so many good things: fibre, low-fat protein and 'good' carbs that deliver nutrients while taking their time going through the digestive system. And they are a snap to incorporate into salads and soups to up the protein quotient. Chickpeas, lentils, navy beans, black beans, kidney beans – there's a bean for every day of the week. But watch out for tinned baked beans with meat, which are high in sugar and fat, and avoid tinned bean soups, which are processed to the point where their overall Gi rating is too high. Homemade bean soups, however, are an excellent choice. You will find several delicious recipes using beans in the recipes section of this book.

Tofu

You don't have to be vegetarian to enjoy tofu, which is low in saturated fat and an excellent source of protein. While tofu is not necessarily a thriller on its own, it takes on the flavours of whatever seasonings and sauces it is cooked with. Seasoned tofu scrambles, for instance, are a good substitute for scrambled eggs. Choose soft tofu, which has up to one-third less fat than the firm variety.

Textured vegetable protein (TVP)

This is not a new device for pre-recording TV shows! TVP is a soya alternative to meat that looks a lot like minced beef, and can be used in the same ways – in lasagne, chilli, stir-fries and Bolognese sauce. It's quite tasty and delivers the texture of meat. Our middle son, a vegetarian who has since left the nest, put us on to this adaptable product.

Potatoes, pasta, rice

These carbohydrates should cover only one-quarter of the plate. Remember, with potatoes your first choice is boiled small new potatoes. Most other choices, especially baked potatoes or chips, are red-light. Sweet potatoes are a good lower-Gi food, but since they tend to come in larger sizes, I suggest you save these for Phase II.

Your serving of pasta should make up no more than a quarter of your meal (about 40g [1 ½oz] uncooked) . Remember to use wholemeal or protein-enriched pasta and avoid cream-based sauces. If you have rice, make it 50g (1 ¾oz) of dry rice – basmati, wild, brown or long-grain rice–per serving.

Vegetables

Here you can put the measuring cup away. Eat as many vegetables and as much salad as you like; they should be the backbone of your meal. Always include at least two vegetables, and remember to cook them just until tender-crisp.

Experiment with something you've never had before. Baby pak choi is delicious grilled, and rapini, a dark-green vegetable that looks like broccoli with more leaves, is a nice change. The dark, curly green vegetables such as kale are full of good things, including folic acid.

Greens such as baby spinach come conveniently pre-washed in bags. Frozen bags of mixed vegetables are also convenient and inexpensive; you can even toss the veggies into a saucepan, add tomato juice with a dollop of salsa and you have a quick vegetable soup.

Dessert

Yes, dessert is part of the Gi Diet – at least, the kind that is green-light and good for you. This includes most fruits, and low-fat dairy products, such as yoghurt and ice cream sweetened with sugar substitute rather than sugar. All my books have recipes for delicious green-light desserts.

Snacks

Keep your digestive system busy and your energy up with between-meal snacks – four a day during the Preliminary Phase and three a day during Phase I. Try to eat balanced snacks that include a bit of protein and carbohydrates; for example, a piece of fruit with a few nuts, or cottage cheese with celery sticks.

A convenient snack for when you're on the go is half a nutrition bar. Be careful when choosing one: most are full of cereal and sugar. The ones to look for contain 20–30g of carbohydrates, 12–15g of protein and 5g of fat. A good green-light choice is Slim-Fast (half a bar per serving).

Keep in mind that many snacks and desserts labelled 'low fat' or 'sugar free' aren't necessarily green-light. Sugar-free instant puddings and 'low-fat' muffins are still high-Gi because they contain highly processed grains.

SNACKS	Red	Yellow	Green
	Bagels	Bananas	Almonds*
	Biscuits	Dark chocolate (70% cocoa)	Apple sauce (unsweetened)
	Chips	Ice cream (low-fat)	Cottage cheese (fat free)
	Crackers	Most nuts	Extra-low-fat cheese (e.g. Laughing Cow Light, Boursin Light)
	Crisps	Popcorn (air-popped)	
	Doughnuts		
	Flavoured jelly (all varieties)		Food bars*
	Ice cream		Fruit yoghurt (non fat with sugar substitute)
	Muffins		
	Popcorn (regular)		Hazelnuts**
	Pretzels		Homemade green-light snacks (see pages 181–204)
	Puddings		
	Raisins		Ice cream (low fat and no added sugar)
	Rice cakes		
	Sorbet		Most fresh fruit
	Tortilla chips		Most fresh vegetables
	Trail mix		Peaches tinned in juice or water
	Sweets		
	White bread		Pears tinned in juice or water
			Pickles
			Pumpkin seeds
			Sugar-free sweets
			Sunflower seeds

* 180–225 calorie bars, e.g. Slim-Fast; ½ bar per serving.
** Limit serving size (see Page 17).

What do I drink?

Because liquids don't trip our satiety mechanisms, it's a waste to take in calories through them. Also, many beverages are high in calories. Juice, for example, is a processed product, and has a much higher Gi than the fruit or vegetable it is made from. A glass of orange juice contains nearly two and a half times the calories of a fresh orange! So eat the fruit or vegetable rather than drink its juice. That way you'll get all the benefits of its nutrients and fibre while consuming fewer calories. As well, stay away from any beverage that contains added sugar or caffeine. As I explained earlier, caffeine stimulates insulin, which leads to us feeling hungry. So no coffee or soft drinks containing caffeine in Phase I.

That said, fluids are an important part of any diet (I'm sure you're all familiar with the eight-glasses-a-day prescription). The following are your best green-light choices.

Water

The cheapest, easiest and best thing to drink is plain water. Seventy per cent of our body consists of water, which is needed for digestion, circulation, regulation of body temperature, lubrication of joints and healthy skin. We can live for months without food, but we can survive only a few days without water.

Don't feel you have to drink eight glasses of water a day in addition to other beverages. Milk, tea and soft drinks all contribute to the eight-glasses-a-day recommendation. But do try to drink a glass of water before each meal – it will help you feel fuller so that you don't overeat.

Skimmed milk

After a sceptical start, I've grown to really enjoy skimmed milk, and I like to drink it with breakfast and lunch, which tend to be a little short on protein. Skimmed milk is an ideal green-light food.

Soft drinks

If you're used to drinking soft drinks, you can still enjoy the sugar- and caffeine-free diet ones. People often treat regular soft drinks and fruit juices as non-foods, but this is how extra calories slip by us.

Tea

Although black and green teas do contain caffeine, the amount is only about one-third of that of coffee. Tea has health benefits as well. Black and green teas contain antioxidant properties that help prevent heart disease and Alzheimer's.

In fact, tea has more flavonoids (antioxidants) than any vegetable tested. Two cups of black or green tea have the same amount of antioxidants as 7 cups of orange juice or 28 cups of apple juice!

So tea in moderation is fine – minus the sugar and cream, of course. Try some new varieties: Darjeeling, Earl Grey, English Breakfast or spicy chai (with sugar substitute). Herbal teas, as long as they are caffeine free, are also a green-light option, though they lack the flavonoids. Iced tea is acceptable if it's sugar free.

Alcohol

Alcohol is generally a disaster for any weight-loss programme. It puts your blood sugar on a roller-coaster: you go up and feel great, then come down and feel like having another drink, or eating the whole bowl of peanuts. Alcohol also contains a lot of calories. So in Phase I, put away the corkscrew and the ice-cube tray. Now that you know how the Gi Diet works, it's time to get ready to start. In the next chapter, I'll outline the steps for launching you into the programme.

TO SUM UP

1. In the Preliminary Phase and Phase I, eat only green-light foods.

2. Eat three balanced meals plus four snacks a day in the Preliminary Phase and three balanced meals plus three snacks in Phase I.

3. Pay attention to portion size: palm of your hand for protein, and a quarter plate for pasta, potatoes or rice. Use common sense and eat moderate amounts.

4. Drink plenty of fluids, including a glass of water with meals and snacks (but no caffeine or alcohol).

4

Before You Start

The Gi Diet is not so much a diet as a completely new and permanent way of eating. This is without question the most important message of this book. Unfortunately, most people view diets as a short-term change in eating habits that are ditched once weight-loss targets have been achieved. They then revert to their old dietary habits and, not surprisingly, they are soon back to their original weight, or worse.

The Gi Diet is the way you will eat for the rest of your life. The one constant refrain I receive from the tens of thousands of successful readers is that this is a new way of eating that has become a permanent part of their lives. Your motivation to lose weight is high, and with the Gi Diet you now have the action plan that will help you make those unwanted pounds disappear. Still, to be successful, you are going to have to make some significant changes in your life, and the better prepared you are, the better equipped you will be to handle any challenges that may arise. The following six steps will get you off to the best possible start.

1. Go to your doctor

Before starting any major change in your eating patterns, check with your doctor to see if you have any health concerns that could affect your weight-loss plans. As you lose weight, your health will certainly improve, and it will be wonderfully motivating to learn that your blood glucose levels have improved or that your blood pressure has gone down. It may even be possible to change any medications you might be taking for weight-related conditions such as diabetes or high blood pressure.

2. Assess whether it's the right time to start

Are you in the middle of a job change? A major house renovation or move? Is it the week before Christmas or a holiday? Then it's probably not the best time to start a new way of eating. Some life events will make it harder – or even impossible – for you to give the programme the attention it needs or to stick with it. Choose a period when your life is relatively stable and when you have time to learn new eating habits – not when your stress levels are even higher than usual. If your enthusiasm for a new slim you is high and the timing is right, then there's no better moment than the present!

3. Set your weight-loss target

It's important to have a healthy, realistic weight-loss target in mind before starting the programme. A good place to start is the BMI table on pages 18–19, not the glossy pages of a fashion or fitness magazine. Being too thin or too heavy is not good. Your health is at risk if your BMI is below 18.5 or above 25. As a woman, with a lower muscle mass and smaller frame than most men, you might want to target the lower end of the healthy range, say around 22, while men should generally target the higher end. Remember, the BMI tables are only a guide. Some of you, who have been carrying a significant amount of extra weight for a long time, will have developed a stronger skeletal frame and increased muscle mass to support this extra weight, and so a BMI in the low 20s would be unrealistic. If this is the case, you will want to target the higher end of the healthy range.

The other measurement you should concern yourself with is your waist measurement, which is an even better predictor of the state of your health than your weight. Abdominal fat is more than just a weight problem. Recent research has shown that abdominal fat acts almost like a separate organ in the body, except this 'organ' is a destructive one that releases harmful proteins and free fatty acids, increasing your risk of life-threatening conditions, especially heart disease.

If you are female and have a waist measurement of 35" (87.5cm) or more, or are male with a waist measurement of over 37" (92.5cm), you are at risk of endangering your health. Women with a measurement of 37" (92.5cm) or more, and men with a measurement over 40" (100cm) are at serious risk of heart disease, stroke, cancer and diabetes.

So I have your attention now! Make sure that you measure correctly: put a tape measure around your waist just above navel level till it fits snugly, without cutting into your flesh. Do not adopt the walking-down-the-beach-sucking-in-your-stomach stance. Just stand naturally. There's no point in trying to fudge the numbers, because the only person you're kidding is yourself.

Now that you know your BMI and waist measurement, you can set your weight-loss target and know roughly how long it will take you to reach that goal. When you lose weight in a healthy way, you can expect to lose about one pound per week. I say 'about' because most people do not lose weight at a fixed and steady rate. The usual pattern is to lose more at the start of the diet, when you are losing mostly water weight, followed by a series of drops and plateaus. The closer you get to your target weight, the slower your weight loss will be. If you are planning to lose up to 20 per cent of your body weight – for example, if you weigh 11 stone and want to lose two stone – assume this will take you thirty weeks, one pound per week. If you have more than 20 per cent to shed, the good news is that you will lose at a faster rate. This is simply because your larger body requires more calories just to keep operating than someone who is lighter. Still, be prepared for measured results – it took you a while to put on those extra pounds and it will take some time to lose them. Be patient and know that once that weight is gone, it will be gone for ever as you keep it off in Phase II of the programme.

Although I recommend recording your progress, please don't get obsessed with numbers on the scale. Many people find themselves losing inches before they register any weight loss. Clothes start feeling a little looser, and, before you know it, you are down a dress size or getting into your old jeans. Soon, you'll probably have to buy new clothes. My readers often tell me that I should have warned them about the extra cost of refurbishing their wardrobe!

4. Give your kitchen a green-light makeover

Take a good look in your fridge – what do you see? Two jars of mayonnaise, some leftover cheddar and a lot of sugar-laden condiments in jars? Now open the cupboards: what's the biscuit and cracker situation? Now is the time to do an honest evaluation of what you tend to keep on hand. Consult the Complete Gi Diet Food Guide (pages 191–204) and throw out anything that's in the red-light column. Be ruthless. If you always have chips on hand, you will eat them. If you keep packets of crisps around 'for the kids', you can be sure that they won't be the only ones snacking on them. Give the unopened food items and cans to your skinny neighbours or local food bank.

5. Eat before you shop

You know what happens when you drop by the supermarket on your way home from work, famished – before you know it, you've bought the biggest tray of cannelloni ever made. The worst mistake you can make is to go shopping on an empty stomach. You'll only be tempted to fill your shopping trolley with high-Gi, sugar-rich foods.

6. Shop green-light

For those of you who prefer a day-to-day guide to your planning, for each week of the Gi Diet Clinic in Part 2, I provide a complete meal and snack plan and a grocery list. If you'd rather not follow the plan, consult Chapter 3 to get some ideas of what you'd like to have for breakfast, lunch, dinner and snacks during your first week on the Gi Diet; have a look at the Complete Gi Diet Food Guide on pages 191–204; and peruse the recipe section of this book or any of my other books.

Write out a shopping list and head out to the supermarket.

Your first few green-light shopping trips will require a bit more time and attention than usual, as you familiarise yourself with green-light eating and meal planning. But don't worry, before long your new shopping and eating habits will become second nature.

Since it would be impossible to include every brand available in today's enormous supermarkets in the Gi Diet Food Guide, I've listed categories of food rather than individual brands, except in cases where clarification is needed, or there is an especially useful product available. This means that you will have to pay some attention to food labels when comparing brands.

When reading a food label, there are six factors to consider in making the best green-light choice:

Serving size

Is the serving size realistic, or has the manufacturer lowered it to make the calories and fat levels look better than the competition's? When comparing brands, ensure you are comparing the same serving size.

Calories

The product with the least amount of calories is obviously the best choice. Some products flagged as 'low fat' still have plenty of calories, so don't be fooled by the diet-friendly slogans. Calories are calories, whether they come from fat or sugar.

Fat

Look at the amount of fat, which is often expressed as a percentage, say 2 per cent (good) or 20 per cent (forget it). Then check to see what sort of fat it is. You want foods that are low fat, with minimal or no saturated fats and trans fats. Remember that trans fats are often called 'hydrogenated oils' or 'partially hydrogenated oils'.

Fibre

Foods with lots of fibre have a low Gi, so this is an important component. When comparing brands, choose the one with higher fibre.

Sugar

Choose products that are low in sugar. Again, watch for products advertised as 'low fat'. Sometimes companies will quietly bump up the sugar content to make up for any perceived loss of taste. This often happens with yoghurts and cereals. Sugars are sometimes listed as dextrose, glucose, fructose or sucrose; regardless of the form, it's sugar.

Sodium

Sodium (salt) increases water retention, which doesn't help when you are trying to lose weight. It also contributes to premenstrual bloating in women and is a factor in hypertension (high blood pressure). Combine high blood pressure with excess weight and you move up to the front of the risk line for heart disease and stroke. Low-sodium products are therefore preferable.

The recommended daily allowance (RDA) of sodium in the UK is 2,400mg (equivalent to a maximum 6g salt). The current average consumption is 3,600mg sodium (9g salt). As many authorities are now recommending 1,500mg sodium (4g salt), it still goes without saying that most of us could stand to cut back on salt. However, if you have a BMI over 30 and have any blood pressure, circulation or heart problems, you need to be even more vigilant about seeking out low-sodium brands. Canned foods like soups are often very high in sodium, as are many fast foods.

You've talked to your doctor, decided there's no better time than the present to lose weight and get healthy, set your weight-loss target, cleared your kitchen of fat-building foods, and restocked your pantry with delicious green-light choices. Now all you have to do is eat green-light meals and snacks each day and you're well on your way to your new trim self. In the next section, you'll find a week-by-week guide to all the challenges and issues that will come up as you follow the Gi Diet for the first thirteen weeks. By the end of it, you will know everything there is to know to achieve your weight-loss dreams, and you'll have lost a significant amount of weight along the way!

TO SUM UP

The six steps to get you launched into the Gi Diet are:

1. Consult your doctor.

2. Assess whether it's the right time in your life to start.

3. Set your weight-loss target.

4. Give your kitchen a green-light makeover.

5. Eat before you shop.

6. Shop green-light.

Week 1 Getting Started

Welcome to Week 1 of the Gi Diet!

You are starting on a journey, a new way of eating that will be the way you eat for the rest of your life. You will never have to go hungry or feel deprived. You won't have to count a calorie or a point. As long as you eat exclusively from the long list of green-light foods in the Complete Gi Diet Food Guide, the extra weight will come off, and you will feel healthy and energetic eating the nutritious green-light way. No more yo-yo dieting! This is the way to lose weight permanently. The first thing I would like you to do is fill in your current measurements below as well as your target weight, so that you have a baseline with which to compare your progress and a place to remind yourself of your ultimate weight-loss goal. There is nothing more motivating than recording your success, so I will be asking you to write down your weight and waist and hip measurements at the end of each week. Be sure to weigh and measure yourself at the same time of day each week, since a meal or even a bowel movement can make a difference of a pound or two at a time when every pound counts! An ideal time is first thing in the morning, before breakfast.

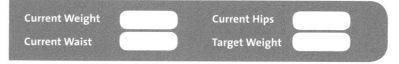

| Current Weight | | Current Hips | |
| Current Waist | | Target Weight | |

Why do you want to lose weight?

Over the next thirteen weeks, I will be providing you with the knowledge, the tools and the counsel to help make this an easy and relatively painless transition to a new way of eating. But ultimately, for the programme to work, you have to want to make it happen and you have to make the commitment to yourself. Whether you want to lose seven pounds or seven stone, it's important to look at the reasons you want to lose weight. Your answer will have a lot to do with your motivation to start and, more important, stay the course with your new way of eating.

The following are some reasons e-Clinic participants gave for wanting to lose weight:

'I am probably seven stone overweight, have high blood pressure, and am facing knee-replacement surgery within the next two years. Time to get serious!' – Karen

'I am a 49-year-old woman who is not aging well ... I am always short of breath and my legs ache constantly. I was recently referred to a gastroenterologist because my blood work showed higher than normal liver enzyme counts. With a warning of the seriousness of a fatty liver, I left feeling so depressed ... I am afraid now for my life.' – Beverley

'I have been heavy all my life ... I remember the jokes and taunting, no proms, no dates ... I am an emotional eater and food has always been my comfort in times of sorrow, distress or loneliness.' – Kathy

'I'm at a point in my life where I have to do something to reduce my weight and improve my health. Perimenopause is giving me some serious problems and I understand that extra weight changes hormone production (and many other things). I am quite certain that returning to an appropriate BMI would decrease the problems I'm having. It's affecting not only my life, but my children's lives and I'm scared for their future. If our family lifestyle changes because I am changing mine, then so much the better. I want and need to do this.' – Cecile

'I am a nurse who should be looking healthy and promoting a healthy lifestyle. I know that the fat that is presently around my waist is not only unattractive but unhealthy. I know that my knees would appreciate me carrying less weight.' – Marcia

'I am a blind person who has put on too much weight over the last few years. For many years, I weighed nine and a half stone. After the death of my parents, I found myself eating chocolate bars in the middle of the night after having numerous nightmares. The weight continued to increase and before I knew it, I am at the weight that I am now. My energy has declined and my old clothes don't fit right. I feel that just because one does not have any vision, that doesn't mean that one should look bad.' – P

'I have always had a weight problem, though not to the extreme, but now, as I am getting older, I have noticed that my hips are sore and I don't have as much energy as I used to. Having four grandsons under five, I want to get myself in better shape to keep up with them.' – Pam

'I know that you often read that one's appearance should not be the motivator but it does help me to envision this time next year, walking into a store and being able to buy a 'regular sized' dress for the holidays.' – Bernadette

Actually, there is absolutely nothing wrong with appearance being a motivator to lose weight. In fact, it is one of the top reasons people want to slim down. Let's look at the three most common reasons people want to lose weight and see how they reflect your own.

1. I want to look better

Judging from the correspondence I have received – 20,000 e-mails and counting – the day when people discover that they have to dig out their 'skinny' pants again is at least as rewarding as seeing the numbers fall on the scale. Most of us would rather shop for clothes that flatter and show off the body rather than resort to camouflage. It's a powerful motivator to walk into a room and hear a friend ask, 'Have you lost weight? You look terrific.' I've sold more books based on word of mouth – people asking Gi Diet readers how they lost their weight – than through any other marketing strategy.

But losing weight is not just about trying to live up to unreachable, red-carpet standards of beauty or thinness; it's about feeling at ease in your body and liking what you see in the mirror. Weight loss boosts self-esteem and confidence, which in turn makes it easier to maintain new eating habits. It's amazing the difference the loss of just a few pounds can make, not only to how you look in your clothes but to how you feel about yourself.

2. I want to feel more energetic and less lethargic

Perhaps what I hear about most frequently from readers, other than the thrill of losing pounds or going down a dress size, is the surge of energy that comes with a lighter, healthier body. Just the other day, I witnessed a dramatic demonstration of the kind of burden extra weight can be. My wife and I had just completed some house renovations to suit our empty-nest lifestyle, and as we were restoring some order, I asked Ruth to carry a couple of 20-pound dumb-bells up a flight of stairs to my new workout room. She could get them only to the first-floor landing before she had to put them down again. 'How do people who are three stone overweight get around, let alone climb stairs?' she wondered. And three stone of extra weight is not something you can just put down when you want to. Imagine the energy that goes into carrying those pounds! That's the energy that will be available to you again if you shed the excess weight.

Readers also tell me about the delight they experience when they find themselves able to do more exercise and to enjoy activities they haven't participated in since their teens. If regaining your former energy and vitality is important to you, you'll receive constant motivation as your new, lighter body rejoices in its recently acquired freedom to run, swim, play squash, or engage in any activity you may have given up for 'lack of energy'.

3. I want to be healthier

Excess weight and poor diet are by far the most critical factors in increasing your chances of developing major diseases that can either undermine your quality of life or drastically shorten it. These include heart disease, stroke, cancer, diabetes and Alzheimer's. Of course, genes play a role in your risk of these diseases too, but anyone who is overweight and undernourished is putting her- or himself at increased risk. The prospect of a long life, especially one free of pain, disability and disease, is a powerful motivator.

Below, I would like you to write down your own personal top three reasons for wanting to lose weight. Take a moment to be clear about your reasons and be absolutely honest – this is for your eyes only. Later on, being able to come back to this page and read what you've written will go a long way towards keeping you motivated and helping you stick to your resolve.

My Top Three Reasons for Losing Weight

1.
2.
3.

Feeling a little nervous?

During the first week of the e-Clinic, everyone got off to an enthusiastic start. However, some participants felt a little trepidation:

'I am afraid and nervous because nothing has worked in the past and it all seems an impossibility now. However, I am committed and will take one day at a time.' – Lynn

'I am anxious to start this new programme. I look forward to the end result which is a slimmer me. I have attempted many other diets but I have failed.' – P

It's perfectly understandable if you're feeling anxious about whether you'll succeed on the Gi Diet, particularly if you've tried and failed on diets before. But please, don't be nervous. I have a file of literally thousands of people who have had great success on the Gi Diet because the programme addresses the very reasons other diets fail. The fact is that most diets really don't work. Why? I'm sure the following explanations will be familiar to you.

Why most diets don't work

1. Most diets leave you feeling hungry, weak and deprived. You stagger through the day with a grumbling stomach but, sooner or later, you cave in and order a pizza with double cheese. Feeling perpetually hungry is the primary reason that people give up on their diet.

2. The diet is too complicated and time-consuming to follow. You spend each day weighing and measuring food, calculating carbs or calories, and keeping food diaries. Perhaps this is fun initially, but then it all just becomes a burden. You're too busy to follow a diet that feels more like a maths exam.

3. You feel bad. Many diets cut out essential nutrients, leaving you feeling lethargic and concerned about your health. No wonder people give up!

Goals and rewards

Feeling nervous about the challenges ahead could be related to the prospect of a long journey and a considerable amount of weight to lose. If so, set a series of mini-goals for yourself. Perhaps your first mini-goal could be to lose one and a half stone, or to break the fourteen-stone barrier, or even to eat perfectly green-light for an entire week.

Decide what your first mini-goal will be and what you will reward yourself with once you reach that goal: a pedicure or a massage? An evening out to a movie or that new book you've been wanting to read? Once you've reached that mini-goal, give yourself a big pat on the back and the reward you promised yourself, and then set your next mini-goal. Setting smaller goals for yourself and reaching them will bolster your self-confidence and convince you of your ability to reach your target weight.

Suffering withdrawal symptoms?

During Week 1, a few participants reported feeling some unpleasant symptoms:

'I am finding that I am having really bad headaches since I have stopped having coffee. Up until Saturday, I would have an extra-large coffee on the way to work. I was in horrible pain today.' – Tammy

'I find I am shaky and light-headed but I am not overly hungry. It is just an awful weak feeling. My hands actually shake and I feel sick. Could this be sugar withdrawal?' – Beverley

Any major change in eating patterns requires an adjustment period, particularly when those high-sugar, high-Gi foods are suddenly dropped from the menu. The good news is that this period of adjustment will be short because the Gi Diet is geared to stabilise blood-sugar levels, preventing those sugar highs and lows that have been a principal contributor to your weight problems.

Getting through the first week will be the hardest part. Drinking just one cup of coffee a day can cause a dependence, as can caffeinated tea or soft drinks. When you suddenly put an end to your caffeine intake, you are likely to experience a headache, fatigue, a 'blue' mood or irritability, and difficulty concentrating. While these symptoms will soon pass, you may want to gradually reduce your caffeine intake, replacing half your regular coffee with decaf, and then making the transition to decaf only. However, if you can't imagine life without your morning jolt of java, go ahead and have it, but make it just one cup a day, and use skimmed milk and sweetener rather than cream and sugar.

By the end of the first week, you will begin to feel much better – even better than you did before you started the Gi Diet, as Ross discovered:

'I stopped drinking coffee and cut out all junk food and junk snacks. Once the withdrawal symptoms passed, I started to feel more energetic ... I've lost 1½ inches from my waist and butt, and 1 inch from my neck. A slightly different guy (second chin shrinking) looks back at me as I shave in front of the morning mirror ... This programme looks fantastic and realistic. For the first time ever, I feel I really can do this.'

A week later, Beverly would write:

'I feel much better than last week when I wrote about the shakes and feeling weak. I actually wake up without a headache – something that has not happened in a long time.'

Congratulate yourself for getting through the first week on the programme, and record your measurements below. Also, take the time to write about your experiences and feelings this week. Diaries help reveal issues you might have to work on, ways of thinking that might be holding you back, or strategies that could work well for you.

Week 1 Diary

Week 1 Weight		Week 1 Waist		Week 1 Hips	

Optional week 1 meal plan

You are not required to use these weekly meal planners and shopping lists. Feel free to pick and choose or make your own green-light meals.

	Breakfast	Snack	Lunch
Mon	Homey Porridge (page 145) with chopped apple	Cranberry Cinnamon Bran Muffin (page 181)	Open-face Chicken Breast sandwich with lettuce, tomato and onion, and Basic Gi Salad (page 153)
Tue	Mini Breakfast Puffs (page 147)	Fruit yoghurt	Gi Pasta Salad (page 156)
Wed	Homemade Muesli (page 145) with skimmed milk and fruit yoghurt	Cranberry Cinnamon Bran Muffin (page 181)	½ wholemeal pitta with canned light tuna, lettuce, tomato and cucumber, and Basic Gi Salad (page 153)
Thu	Homey Porridge (page 145) with berries	Small apple and a glass of skimmed milk	Quick and Easy Chicken Noodle Soup (page 151) and Basic Gi Salad (page 153)
Fri	All-Bran with skimmed milk, peach slices and sliced almonds	Fruit yoghurt	Mixed Bean Salad (page 157)
Sat	Western Omelette (page 149) or Homey Porridge (page 145)	½ food bar	Greek Salad (page 155)
Sun	Oatmeal Buttermilk Pancakes with Strawberries (page 146)	Orange and almonds	Tuscan White Bean Soup (page 151) and Basic Gi Salad (page 153)

Week 1 shopping list for meal plan

Produce

Almonds (whole and sliced)
Apples
Asparagus
Aubergines
Baby spinach
Bean sprouts
Blueberries or mixed summer berries (fresh or frozen)
Broccoli
Carrots
Celery
Courgettes
Cranberries (dried)
Cucumbers
Fresh herbs (chives, mint, flat-leaf parsley, sage, tarragon, thyme)
Garlic
Green beans
Kale
Leeks
Lemons
Lettuce (iceberg, leaf and Cos)
Mixed nuts
Mushrooms
Onions (yellow and red)
Oranges
Peaches (fresh or tinned in juice or water)
Peppers (red and green)
Potatoes (new, small)
Plums

Snack	Dinner	Snack
Laughing Cow Light cheese with high-fibre crispbread	Easy-Bake Lasagne (page 163) and Caesar salad	Mixed berries tossed in lime juice with soured cream
Hummus with carrot and celery sticks	Gi Fish Fillet (page 166), asparagus, carrots and new potatoes	Orange and almonds
Cottage cheese (low-fat) with peach slices	Chicken Curry (page 170), and Raita Salad (page 152)	Apple Pie Cookie (page 188), and glass of skimmed milk
Crunchy Chickpeas (page 181)	Vegetable Crumble (page 161) and Tabbouleh Salad (page 156)	½ food bar
Laughing Cow Light cheese with high-fibre crispbread	Chicken Fried Rice (page 170)	Mixed berries tossed in lime juice with soured cream
Hummus with carrot and celery sticks	Beef and Aubergine Chilli (page 176) and Basic Gi Salad (page 153)	Apple Pie Cookie (page 188) and a glass of skimmed milk
Fruit yoghurt	Pork Medallions Dijon (page 178), green beans, carrots and new potatoes	Piece of Plum Crumble (page 186)

Raisins
Sesame seeds
Spring onions
Strawberries
Sunflower seeds (shelled, unsalted)
Sweet potato
Tofu (firm)
Tomatoes (plum)

Deli
Feta cheese (light)
Hummus (light)
Kalamata olives
Parmesan cheese, grated

Bakery
100% stone-ground wholemeal bread

High-fibre crispbread
Wholemeal pitta bread

Fish counter
Fish fillets (salmon or trout)

Meat counter
Back bacon
Beef mince (extra-lean)
Chicken breasts (boneless, skinless)
Pork tenderloins

Beans (legumes) and tinned vegetables
Chickpeas
Kidney beans (red and white)
Mixed beans
Tomatoes (chopped)

Tomatoes (plum)
Tomato puree

Pasta and sauces
Fusilli or Penne (wholemeal)
Lasagne (wholemeal)
Light tomato sauce (no added sugar)
Low-fat pasta sauce (no cheese or meat in sauce)
Small-shaped pasta (e.g. ditali or tubetti)

Soup and tinned seafood and meat
Anchovy fillets
Chicken stock (low fat, low salt)
Tuna (light, in water)
Vegetable stock (low fat, low salt)

Grains and side dishes
Basmati rice
Brown rice
Bulgur wheat
Flaxseeds (ground)

International foods
Sesame oil
Soy sauce (low salt)
Tahini

Cooking oil, vinegar, salad dressings and pickles
Cooking oil spray (vegetable or olive oil)
Dijon mustard
Mayonnaise (fat-free)
Oil (vegetable and extra-virgin olive)
Red wine vinegar
Worcestershire sauce

Snacks
Apple sauce (unsweetened)
Food bars (e.g. Slim-Fast)

Baking
Baking powder
Bicarbonate of soda
Cornflour
Oat bran
Spices (ground cardamom, cayenne pepper, chilli powder, ground cinnamon, ground cumin, curry powder, ground ginger, ground nutmeg, dried oregano, black pepper, red-pepper flakes, salt, dried thyme)
Splenda
Vanilla extract
Wheat bran
Wheat germ
Wholemeal flour

Breakfast foods
All-Bran cereal
Oatmeal (large-flake oats)

Beverages
White wine

Dairy
Buttermilk
Cheddar (low fat)
Cottage cheese (low fat)
Fruit yoghurt (non-fat with sweetener)
Laughing Cow cheese (light)
Margarine (soft, non-hydrogenated, light)
Milk (skimmed)
Mozzarella cheese (low fat)
Plain yoghurt (non-fat)
Soured cream (light)
Whole Omega-3 eggs

Frozen foods
Mixed berries
Peas

Week 2 Meal Planning

This week, I want to talk to you about meal planning and shopping. Setting some time aside each week to plan your meals and snacks for the seven days ahead is one of the most important things you can do to ensure you eat well and stick to the programme, as many of our e-Clinic participants discovered:

'I've learned there is much truth to the saying "failing to plan is planning to fail". In light of that, I prepared four selections from your cookbook last night to eat this week. Oh my goodness, the yoghurt cheese with the sweetener and orange zest is fabulous! I made the almond-encrusted pears and put them (along with the yoghurt cheese) on my oatmeal this morning ... it was delicious. I also made the lentil and garbanzo bean salad, the chicken enchiladas, and the lentil and brown rice-stuffed peppers. So I'm going into the week prepared with some really yummy and healthy foods!' – Nancy

'Well, I am embarrassed about what a bad week it has been. I was not prepared for many really busy days and I have subsequently made poor choices daily. The whole week was just one problem perpetuating another. I have told you in the past that I do feel physically better when I make better food choices, but at a time when I needed as much energy as possible, I made the worst choices. So, this week, I am going to try a combination of better advance planning and writing down what I eat. I am trying not to feel too discouraged, as I really want to see success with this approach, but this week has shown me that determination alone is not sufficient if you don't make other changes also.' – Bernadette

'I had a much better week. Prior planning is the key so that snacks are ready and available. A shopping plan and list has solved this problem. Also brown-bagging it is so much easier. I bought an insulated nylon lunch bag with tons of room – works great.' – Ross

'I plan my meals in advance for a week due to my long commute and adjust as necessary.' – Kathy

By and large, participants found that planning ahead was key to their success on the programme. If they neglected to do it, they tended to grab whatever happened to be easily available – and it usually wasn't green-light! Knowing what you are going to be eating each day and having all the ingredients at hand will not only ensure that you eat right, but also make your life simpler and put your mind at ease. This is why I have provided a green-light meal plan and shopping list for each week. I realise that some people enjoy cooking and trying new recipes, while others do not, and so these meal plans might not be practical for everyone. By the end of the thirteen weeks of the e-Clinic, Ross and Bernadette had found a meal-planning strategy that worked best for them:

'For many weeks, I struggled with the feeling that I had to start making full meals, and felt some (internal) pressure to start using recipes. But a simple approach to food preparation is working well for me and my family, and the foods we are having may be somewhat plain by other people's standards, but so what? Fresh, homemade foods that are naturally tasty and colourful are working well for us. So we will stick to this for now.' – Bernadette

'I now work out a plan for a week or so, listing the days and the meals and a possible "menu" – nothing fancy – for example, seven breakfasts, six lunches, and six dinners to cover before the next grocery trip. Then I calculate roughly what I will need for these meals by total breakfasts, lunches, dinners, snacks – not by specific days, that's far too anal for me. This only takes a few minutes to actually do the "math" and write the list plus of course actually do the shopping. Say, seven breakfasts equals oatmeal for five, high-fibre cereal for two, milk, sugar substitute, so many pieces of toast, jam, fruit etc. I calculate what I want for this meal period and timeframe and buy what I need to bring the "in home" stock up to cover this meal period so I have no excuse to run out to Tim's because I need breakfast but don't have time to go shopping right now.' – Ross

Decide what will work best for you in terms of meal planning and shopping, and then make your health a priority by following through.

Turning your standbys into green-light recipes
You don't necessarily have to use all the recipes in this book; in fact, you can make many of your own standbys green-light by following the guidelines below.

Green-light ingredients
First, ensure that all the ingredients in the recipe are green-light. If there are any red- or yellow-light ingredients, either omit them or replace them with a green-light alternative. Some red- and yellow-light foods can be used in recipes if there is a very limited quantity, such as 125ml wine in a dish that will serve six people, or 4tbsp raisins in a salad for four people. Full-flavoured cheeses can also be used sparingly occasionally. For example, a tablespoon or two of grated Parmesan cheese sprinkled over a casserole will add flavour without too many calories. As long as the red- and yellow-light ingredients are used in limited quantities and not as a core ingredient, they will not have a significant impact on the overall Gi or green-light rating of the recipe.

Fibre

The fibre content of the recipe is critical. Fibre, both soluble and insoluble, is key to the overall Gi rating of a recipe. The more, the better. If your recipe is light on fibre then consider adding fibre boosters such as oats, bran, whole grains or beans.

Fat

The recipe should be low in fat with little to no saturated fat. If fat is called for, use vegetable oil. Olive oil is your best choice, but as little as possible as all fats are calorie dense.

Sugar

Never add sugar or sugar-based ingredients such as corn syrup or molasses. There are some excellent sugar substitutes on the market. Our favourite is Splenda, or sucralose, which was developed from a sugar base but does not have the calories. It works well in cooking and baking. Measure it by volume (not weight) to exactly replace sugar. For example, 1 tablespoon sugar = 1 tablespoon Splenda. Note that Brown Splenda is 50 per cent sugar and is therefore not recommended.

Protein

Confirm that the recipe contains sufficient protein, or that you are serving it alongside some protein to round out the meal. Protein helps slow the digestive process, which effectively lowers the Gi of a recipe. It is also the one component that is often overlooked, particularly in recipes for salads and snacks. Useful protein boosters are low-fat dairy products; lean meats, poultry and seafood; egg whites; beans; and soya-based foods such as tofu and isolated soy or whey powders.

Maximising the time you spend cooking

If you don't always have time to cook, make big batches when you do have time, say on the weekends, and freeze green-light meals for busy nights. Having healthy meals in your freezer means you can always pull them out rather than grab a take-away menu. With a little preplanning, you won't have to rely on fast food to get you through your busy schedule! Organizing your pantry, fridge and freezer so that they keep you going when the going gets tough will ensure the weight-loss results you want, as Karen learned this week:

'My weight is probably skewed because I have had bronchitis. Believe me, the combination of codeine, amoxicillin and cough drops is more effective than any diet I've ever been on! I am sure that once I get back to eating regularly, my weight will go up, or at least I won't see any loss. Please remind me of this next week when I am discouraged. On the bright side, since I had already cleaned out my pantry and fridge, I didn't have my typical "woe is me" feast of grilled cheese, tomato soup, and chocolate ice cream/brownies.' – Karen

Week 2 Weight		Week 2 Waist		Week 2 Hips	

Week 2 Diary

_____

_____

_____

_____

_____

_____

_____

_____

_____

Optional week 2 meal plan

	Breakfast	Snack	Lunch
Mon	Homey Porridge (page 145) with chopped apple	Carrot Muffin (page 182)	Open-face lean deli ham sandwich with lettuce, tomato, red pepper and wholegrain mustard, and Basic Gi Salad (page 153)
Tue	Mini Breakfast Puffs (page 147)	Fruit yoghurt	Waldorf Chicken and Rice Salad (page 157)
Wed	Homemade Muesli (page 145) with skimmed milk and fruit yoghurt	Carrot Muffin (page 182)	Cottage cheese with apple and grapes, and Basic Gi Salad (page 153)
Thu	Homey Porridge (page 145) with blueberries	Small apple and a glass of skimmed milk	Minestrone Soup, Basic Gi Salad (page 153)
Fri	All-Bran with skimmed milk, peach slices and sliced almonds	Fruit yoghurt	½ wholemeal pitta with deli turkey, lettuce, tomatoes and cucumber, and Basic Gi Salad (page 153)
Sat	Italian Omelette (page 148) or Homey Porridge (page 145)	½ food bar	Crab Salad in Tomato Shells (page 158)
Sun	Cinnamon French Toast (page 146) with back bacon	Orange and almonds	Ham and Lentil Soup (page 152) and Basic Gi Salad (page 153)

Snack	Dinner	Snack
Laughing Cow Light cheese with high-fibre crispbread	Fettuccine Primavera (page 159) and Caesar Salad (page 154)	Mixed berries tossed in lime juice with soured cream
Hummus with carrot and celery sticks	Ginger-Wasabi Halibut (page 167), Cold Noodle Salad with Cucumber and Sesame (page 155), snow peas and carrots	Orange and almonds
Fruit yoghurt	Chicken Tarragon with Mushrooms (page 173), broccoli and basmati rice	Pecan Brownie (page 189) and a glass of skimmed milk
Crunchy Chickpeas (Page 181)	Meatloaf (page 175), green beans, carrots and new potatoes	1/2 food bar
Laughing Cow Light cheese with high-fibre crispbread	Bean and Onion Pizza (page 162)	Mixed berries tossed in lime juice with soured cream
Hummus with carrot and celery sticks	Grilled Tuna with Chimichurri Sauce (page 168), asparagus and new potatoes	Pecan Brownie (page 189) and a glass of skimmed milk
Yoghurt with peach slices	Orange Chicken with Almonds (page 172), green beans and basmati rice	Slice of Apple Raspberry Coffee Cake (page 187)

Week 2 shopping list for meal plan

Produce
Almonds (whole and sliced)
Apples
Asparagus
Baby spinach
Blueberries or mixed summer berries
(fresh or frozen)
Broccoli
Carrots
Celery
Courgettes
Cucumbers
Fresh herbs (basil, chives, coriander,
flat-leaf parsley)
Garlic
Ginger root
Grapes
Green beans
Lemon
Lettuce (leaf and Cos)
Limes
Mangetout
Mushrooms
Onions (yellow and red)
Oranges
Peaches (fresh or tinned in juice or
water)
Pecans
Peppers (red and green)
Potatoes (new, small)
Raisins
Raspberries
Sesame seeds
Spring onions
Strawberries
Sunflower seeds, shelled and
unsalted
Tofu (firm)
Tomatoes (large beefsteak and plum)
Tomatoes (sun-dried)
Walnuts

Deli
Feta cheese (low fat)
Hummus
Lean deli ham
Lean deli turkey
Parmesan cheese, grated

Bakery
High-fibre crispbread
100% stone-ground wholemeal
bread
Wholemeal pitta bread

Fish
Frozen crab
Halibut fillets
Tuna steaks (1/2-inch thick)

Meat
Back bacon
Chicken breasts (boneless, skinless)
Minced beef (extra-lean)

Beans (legumes) and canned vegetables
Chickpeas
Kidney beans (red and white)
Lentils
Tomatoes (plum)
Tomato purée

Pasta and sauces
Capellini or spaghetti (wholemeal)
Fettuccine or linguine (wholemeal)
Low-fat pasta sauce (no cheese or
meat in sauce)
Small-shaped pasta (ditali or tubetti)

Soup and canned seafood and meat
Anchovy fillets
Basmati rice
Chicken stock (low fat, low salt)
Vegetable stock (low fat, low salt)

Grains and side dishes
Flaxseeds (ground)

International foods
Mirin (or sweet sherry)
Rice vinegar
Sesame seeds (toasted)
Soy sauce (low salt)
Tahini
Wasabi powder

Cooking oil, vinegar, salad dressings and pickles
Buttermilk salad dressing (low fat, low sugar)
Cooking oil spray (vegetable or olive oil)
Dijon mustard
Oil (vegetable and extra-virgin olive)
Red wine vinegar
Wholegrain mustard
Worcestershire sauce

Snacks
Food bars (e.g. Slim-Fast)

Baking
Active dry yeast
Baking powder
Bicarbonate of soda
Brown-sugar substitute
Cornflour
Oat bran

Spices (black pepper, cayenne pepper, ground cinnamon, ground ginger, ground nutmeg, dried oregano, red-pepper flakes, salt, dried tarragon, dried thyme)
Splenda
Unsweetened cocoa powder
Vanilla extract
Wheat bran
Wheat germ
Wholemeal flour

Breakfast foods
All-Bran cereal
Oatmeal (large-flake oats)

Beverages
Tomato juice
Vegetable cocktail juice
Vermouth or white wine

Dairy
Buttermilk
Fruit yoghurt (non-fat with sweetener)
Laughing Cow cheese (Light)
Margarine (soft, non-hydrogenated, light)
Milk (skimmed)
Mozzarella cheese (part skimmed)
Soured cream (low fat)
Whole Omega-3 eggs

Frozen foods
Peas (or fresh)
Mixed berries

Week 3 Behaviour Change

This week was clearly a period of adjustment as e-Clinic participants came to terms with the day-to-day realities of changing their eating habits:

'Finishing things the kids have left on their plates has become such an established habit for me that there were times I was shocked to see myself on 'autopilot' just doing this, completely unrelated to being hungry.' – Bernadette

'I had a good week but found that eating breakfast is the hardest thing for me to do. I am not really hungry, so I am choking down high-fibre cereal at my desk at seven in the morning. The weekend was better because I had time to make oatmeal, and you are right, it stays with you a lot longer than anything else.' – Beverley

'I found out that, for me, nuts can't be a snack. It is too easy to take a handful of cashews and almonds rather than the suggested amount, or to pop one or two extra as I count out the correct amount.' – Kathy

'I think where I went wrong this week was not eating enough small snacks. As a matter of fact, I often skipped the snacks thinking that would help me in the long run ... and more weight would be lost. Boy, I sure got fooled.' – P

'My problem is that I get really busy and forget to eat until I am starved and would eat any and everything in my sight. I know this is not the way to be successful but will work on eating and snacking at the right times.' – Carol

'Weekends are the hardest for me as I don't have the structure of my workday with break time and lunch, so I may have to resort to a timer or alarm to remind me to eat. I usually end up not eating much at all throughout the day, then realizing I didn't eat very much and then having a slightly larger than normal dinner. I simply forget to eat as I don't feel hungry – I get busy with doing things around the house or out and about and it doesn't occur to me to eat something.' – Kimberley

Kimberley has an excellent idea there! If you are having trouble remembering to eat all your snacks and meals, why not buy a cheap watch with an alarm that you can set to remind yourself to eat? I have one myself for exactly that purpose, though of course it becomes unnecessary after a while when regular eating becomes second nature. Whatever you do, please don't forget to refuel! When you skip snacks or meals, you end up only eating more – not less – by day's end.

Breaking bad habits

Let's face it: change isn't always easy. Old habits can be hard to break. But to lose a significant amount of weight permanently, it is absolutely necessary to ditch old eating habits that led to the weight gain in the first place. Simply modifying your existing way of eating won't do it; you have to rethink your priorities and be willing to make fundamental changes in the way you approach food and eating. Making the commitment to commit is half the battle; making the necessary life changes is the rest. To ease the transition, bad habits will need to be replaced with good habits that you can easily handle. The following is a list of the top ten bad habits that prevent weight loss and what can be done to change them.

1. Skipping Breakfast

This is a very common bad habit. Many people make a habit of skipping breakfast in the morning, but this is a big mistake. By doing so, people leave their stomachs empty from dinner to lunch the next day, often more than sixteen hours! No wonder they overeat at lunch and then look for a sugar fix mid-afternoon as they run out of steam. Breakfast is the most important meal of the day. By the time people rise in the morning, most haven't eaten for ten to twelve hours, and their blood-sugar levels are low. As a result, skipping breakfast will almost certainly cause you to snack throughout the day in an effort to boost your blood-sugar, or energy, level. And chances are good that you will reach for high-calorie, high-fat foods such as doughnuts, muffins or cookies to give you that quick sugar fix your body feels it needs. But as we are all well aware by now, the blood-sugar high caused by these red-light foods will soon be followed by a sugar crash as your insulin kicks in, and you'll be looking for your next sugar fix.

It's tremendously important that you never skip breakfast, and that you spread your daily calorie intake evenly throughout the day. Research consistently shows that people who eat breakfast actually eat fewer calories per day and lose weight more successfully than those who do not. Always start your day with a substantial breakfast.

2. Not taking time to eat properly

Saying 'I don't have time to eat properly' creates a spawning ground for bad habits. People who don't take the time to eat properly tend to grab a coffee and Danish on their way to work, eat a store-bought muffin mid-morning to boost flagging energy levels, have a slice or two of pizza with Coke for lunch, snack on chocolate and cookies in the afternoon to help keep their eyes open, pick up some high-fat takeaway food on the way home for dinner, and, finally, collapse in front of the TV for the evening with a beer and a packet of crisps.

It's easy to slip into this harmful cycle of fattening convenience foods and short-term energy fixes, but you'll pay for the convenience with a growing girth, flagging energy and poor health.

And, really, the amount of incremental time required to prepare your own healthy meals and snacks is quite modest. Fifteen minutes in the morning is all it takes to eat a healthy breakfast – often the length of time it takes to queue at Costa for a coffee. If you can't manage to wake up fifteen minutes earlier to squeeze in a nutritious breakfast before rushing off to work, then bring along a box of green-light cereal, a carton of skimmed milk and a piece of fruit. Another piece of fruit and a carton of skimmed milk takes no time to prepare and makes a filling, nutritious snack. And there are always places where you can get a green-light sandwich so you don't resort to pizza. Eating healthily throughout the day will ensure you have the energy when you arrive home to prepare a quick green-light dinner in the time it would have taken to drive to the take-away and wait for your order. A little extra time and thought is all that's required to break out of the 'I don't have time ...' habits for good.

3. Grazing

The world's best grazers are teenagers. They simply cannot avoid opening the fridge every time they pass it. Their rapid growth and (hopefully) high activity levels require a constant high-calorie intake. Unfortunately, grazing is a habit that many people continue into their adult lives with disastrous results for their waistlines and health. A few nuts here, a couple of cookies there, a tablespoon or two of peanut butter, and a few glasses of juice all look pretty harmless in themselves, but taken together they can easily total several hundred extra calories a day! And those can add up to over one and a half stone of additional weight in a year.

On the Gi Diet, you should be eating three meals plus three to four snacks a day, which means you are eating something approximately every two hours or so during your waking hours. This will reduce your temptation to graze. One reader wrote that she couldn't believe how she could be losing weight when she always seemed to be eating. She called it 'green-light grazing'!

4. Unconscious eating

How often have any of us begun to nibble on a bowl of nuts or crisps or a box of cookies while watching TV, reading a book or talking on the phone and then suddenly realised that we'd eaten the whole lot? Too often, I would guess. Eating should never be the peripheral activity – it should always be the focus. Eat your meals at the table and set aside distractions such as the TV, computer, video game or telephone while you have your snacks. This will help you to always eat consciously and be aware of exactly how much you are eating.

5. Eating too quickly

The famous Dr Johnson of the eighteenth century is said to have asserted that food should always be chewed thirty-two times before swallowing. Though this seems rather excessive, there is an important truth here. Many of us tend to eat far too quickly. It takes twenty to thirty minutes for the stomach to let the brain know it is full. If you eat too quickly, you'll continue to eat past the point at which you've had enough. The solution, then, is to eat slowly to allow your brain to catch up with your stomach.

That's probably another reason Mediterranean countries have lower rates of obesity: they take far longer to eat their meals. There, mealtimes are for family and friends, and for enjoying the pleasure of food – not simply a means to tackle hunger. To ensure you are not eating more than your appetite requires, slow down and really enjoy what you are eating. Put your fork down between mouthfuls. Savour the flavours and textures.

6. Not drinking enough

Did you know that by the time you feel thirsty you are already dehydrated? Your body's need for water is second only to its need for oxygen. Up to 70 per cent of the body is water, and we should be drinking about eight glasses a day to replenish our supply. Yet many of us don't take the time to drink enough, and we go through our days in a mild state of dehydration. Being dehydrated makes us feel tired and hungry, which makes us reach for food when really we should be reaching for a glass of water. Our body isn't hungry, it's thirsty. So always carry a water bottle with you and make sure you are drinking the recommended amount. Being properly hydrated will go a long way towards helping you control your appetite and lose weight.

7. Rewarding for exercise

Another common habit is to reward yourself with food for doing some exercise. Rather than allowing the reward to lie in the exercise itself, many feel that making the extra effort deserves some form of reward or treat, which more often than not takes the form of food or drink.

This raises a couple of issues. First, one of the great myths about weight loss is that it can be achieved through exercise. Though exercise is essential for long-term health and weight maintenance, it is actually a poor tool for losing weight. To give you an idea of how much exercise you would have to do to lose just one pound of fat, you would have to walk briskly for 42 miles if you weighed 11½ stone or 53 miles if you weighed 9 stone. That is a huge amount of effort and way beyond the capabilities or time availability of most people. Walking around the block or washing the car consumes only a handful of calories. So if you are using exercise for permission to cut a little slack in your diet, remember that that cookie reward will add more calories than you expended on your activity.

By all means exercise to improve your health, but don't think it will contribute a whole lot to your weight loss. I frequently tell people that losing weight is 90 per cent diet and 10 per cent exercise, particularly in the early stages.

8. Cleaning the plate

Many of us were taught from the time we were small to finish what's on our plates before leaving the table. This becomes a deeply embedded habit that does not, unfortunately, help us in later life to lose or maintain weight. Not only do we finish our own food, but we also tend to finish the leftovers on our children's plates or that last lonely slice in the pie dish after dinner. I confess that I do this. But this habit causes us to eat more than we need to satisfy our hunger and is therefore dreadful for weight control. Get into the habit of letting your stomach and brain decide when you are full, not the quantity of food on your plate. Leftovers can always be stored in the fridge, rather than around your waist and hips.

9. Shopping on an empty stomach

Human nature can often be perverse, encouraging us to do the right thing but at the wrong time. When you are full and satisfied, food shopping is rarely at the top of your mind. But when you are hungry, grocery shopping suddenly seems like a very good idea indeed. Unfortunately, it just isn't: you'll end up with a shopping trolley that has been filled primarily by your stomach rather than your head. Those red-light foods will seem far more tempting than usual and you will probably make some poor choices as a result. So always shop after a meal, or at least take a green-light snack with you, such as a nutrition bar. You'll make far wiser choices this way.

10. Eating high-sugar, high-fat treats

As we are all well aware, food is a big part of holidays and celebrations – just think of Christmas or a wedding, and you'll probably picture the foods that go along with them. Food is inexorably linked with positive experiences, and that is one reason we often think of certain foods as treats. Whether it's Granny doling out sweets to a child who has been good, or a neighbour presenting you with a freshly baked pie as reward for raking up her leaves, we are accustomed to using food treats to reward the people in our lives as well as ourselves.

Unfortunately, these so-called treats tend to be high in calories, sugar and fat, and are certainly not your friends. They are a major contributor to the obesity crisis and to weight-related diseases like diabetes and heart disease. We should really start to view these foods as penalties rather than rewards.

Instead, choose treats that are lower in calories and fat. If sweets are your thing, there is a plethora of low- and no-sugar brands available. Fresh fruit and low-fat and no-sugar-added yoghurt and ice cream are even better treats. And there are many delicious green-light dessert and snack recipes in all my Gi Diet books.

Keep in mind that while it will take some effort and be challenging at times to change old bad habits, it's well worth your while to persevere with beneficial new behaviours. Before you know it, they'll be second nature, new habits as firmly entrenched as the old ones used to be. But these ones will help you slim down to a brand new you. To end this week on a positive note, here are some observations from e-Clinic participants as they completed Week 3 of the programme:

'It's been a pretty good week ... I've stayed totally on track with my eating, and feel so much better physically (despite being sick) and have much more confidence in my ability to totally adapt to this lifestyle and get to my goal weight.'
– Nancy

'I feel more energetic for sure, and loose pants are still in fashion so I won't need new pants just yet.' Ross

'The weight is coming off so easy, I am really excited.' – Tammy

Week 3 Weight		Week 3 Waist		Week 3 Hips	

Week 3 Diary

Optional week 3 meal plan

	Breakfast	Snack	Lunch
Mon	Homey Porridge (page 145) with chopped apple	Apple Bran Muffin (page 182)	Open-face chicken sandwich with lettuce, tomato and onion and Basic Gi Salad (page 153)
Tue	Mini Breakfast Puffs (page 147)	Fruit yoghurt	Gi Pasta Salad (page 156)
Wed	Homemade Muesli (page 145) with skimmed milk and fruit yoghurt	Apple Bran Muffin (page 182)	½ wholemeal pitta with canned light tuna, lettuce, tomato and cucumber and Basic Gi Salad (page 153)
Thu	Homey Porridge (page 145) with blueberries	Small apple and a glass of skimmed milk	Quick and Easy Chicken Noodle Soup (page 151) and Basic Gi Salad (page 153)
Fri	All-Bran with skimmed milk, peach slices and sliced almonds	Fruit yoghurt	Mixed Bean Salad (page 157)
Sat	Vegetarian Omelette (page 149) or Homey Porridge (page 145)	½ food bar	Greek Salad (page 155)
Sun	Oatmeal Buttermilk Pancakes with Strawberries (page 146)	Orange and almonds	Tuscan White Bean Soup (page 151) and Basic Gi Salad (page 153)

Week 3 shopping list for meal plan

Produce
Almonds (whole and sliced)
Apples
Aubergines
Blueberries or mixed summer berries (fresh or frozen)
Broccoli
Brussels sprouts
Cabbage (green and red)
Carrots
Celery
Courgettes
Cucumbers
Currants
Fresh herbs (chives, coriander, flat-leaf parsley, mint, rosemary, sage and thyme)
Garlic
Green beans

Kale
Leek
Lemons
Lettuce (leaf, iceberg and Cos)
Limes
Mushrooms
Onions (yellow and red)
Oranges
Peaches (fresh or tinned in juice or water)
Pecans
Peppers (red and green)
Potatoes (new, small)
Spring onions
Strawberries
Sunflower seeds, shelled and unsalted
Tomatoes (plum)

Snack	Dinner	Snack
Laughing Cow Light cheese with high-fibre crispbread	Rigatoni with Mini-Meatballs (page 177) and Caesar Salad (page 154)	Mixed berries tossed in lime juice with soured cream
Hummus with carrot and celery sticks	Citrus-Poached Haddock (page 167), green beans and new potatoes	Orange and almonds
Cottage cheese with fruit slices	Chicken Jambalaya (page 172) and broccoli	Creamy Lemon Square (page 190) and a glass of skimmed milk
Crunchy Chickpeas (page 181)	Barley Risotto with Leeks, Lemon and Peas (page 160) and Tabbouleh Salad (page 156)	½ food bar
Laughing Cow Light cheese with high fibre crispbread	Thai Red Curry Prawn Pasta (page 166)	Mixed berries tossed in lime juice with soured cream
Hummus with carrot and celery sticks	Zesty Barbecued Chicken (page 174), Tangy Red and Green Coleslaw (page 153) and new potatoes	Creamy Lemon Square (page 190) and a glass of skimmed milk
Fruit yoghurt	Pork Tenderloin with Apple Compote (page 180), Brussels sprouts, carrots and new potatoes	Piece of Berry Crumble (page 185)

Deli
Feta cheese (light)
Hummus (light)
Kalamata olives
Parmesan cheese, grated

Bakery
100% stone-ground wholemeal bread
High-fibre crispbread
Wholemeal pitta bread

Fish
Haddock fillets
Prawns (large, raw)

Meat
Chicken breasts (boneless, skinless)
Lean chicken or turkey mince
Pork tenderloin

Beans (legumes) and canned vegetables
Chickpeas
Kidney beans (red and white)
Mixed beans
Tomatoes (plum)
Tomatoes (stewed)
Tomato puree

Pasta and sauces
Light tomato sauce
Macaroni or small shells (wholemeal)
Rigatoni (wholemeal)
Fusilli or penne (wholemeal)
Small-shaped pasta (e.g. ditali or tubetti)
Spaghetti or linguine (wholemeal)

Soup and tinned seafood and meat
Anchovy fillets
Chicken stock (low fat, low salt)
Tuna (light, in water)
Vegetable stock (low fat, low salt)

Grains and side dishes
Barley
Brown rice
Bulgur wheat
Flaxseeds (ground)

International foods
Tahini
Thai red curry paste

Cooking oil, vinegar, salad dressings and pickles
Cider vinegar
Cooking oil spray (vegetable or olive oil)
Dijon mustard
Mayonnaise (fat free)
Oil (vegetable and extra-virgin olive)
Red wine vinegar
Worcestershire sauce

Snacks
Apple sauce (unsweetened)
Food bars (e.g. Slim-Fast)

Baking
Baking powder
Bicarbonate of soda
Brown-sugar substitute
Cornflour
Ground almonds
Oat bran

Spices (ground allspice, bay leaves, black pepper, cayenne pepper, celery seeds, chilli powder, ground cinnamon, ground cloves, ground cumin, dried oregano, dried sage, salt and dried thyme)
Splenda
Vanilla extract
Wheat bran
Wheat germ
Wholemeal flour

Breakfast foods
All-Bran cereal
Oatmeal (large-flake oats)

Beverages
Apple juice (unsweetened)
Dry white wine (or vermouth)

Dairy
Buttermilk
Cheddar cheese (low fat)
Cottage cheese (low fat)
Fruit yoghurt (non-fat with sweetener)
Laughing Cow cheese (Light)
Margarine (soft, non-hydrogenated, light)
Milk (skimmed)
Orange juice (unsweetened)
Soured cream (low fat)
Whole omega-3 eggs

Frozen foods
Frozen apple-juice concentrate
Mixed berries
Peas (or fresh)

Week 4 Falling off the Wagon

Falling off the wagon is bound to happen sooner or later. And while I don't encourage it, it's acceptable as long as it's the exception and not the rule. This diet isn't meant to be a straitjacket, after all. If you do your best to eat the green-light way 90 per cent of the time, you'll still lose weight. The odd lapse, at worst, will delay you by a week or two from reaching your target weight. So don't be so hard on yourself, just get right back on the plan with the next meal. Some people make the mistake of feeling so bad about having a slip-up that they just give up. But you should anticipate that you will fall off the wagon from time to time. The best way to handle it is to learn why it happened and decide how you will handle the situation the next time. Rather than dwell on the negative, think about the positive, as Ross did:

'There was a family dinner party with Chinese food where I strayed, but remarkably I only had one medium plate and not the usual two heaping plates of food I would have had in the past. Also, I felt no hunger pains when I didn't have the extra food this time – a definite change.'

Here's how e-Clinic participants dealt with their occasional slip-ups:

'Results while unfortunate were not unexpected. Two of the top three listed side effects of the prednisone I'm taking are increased appetite and weight gain. I've been eating a lot more. At home and the office, I've been limited to green-light foods, but the other day at a restaurant for lunch I found myself eating cornbread! I never eat cornbread. At least I didn't butter it. Two lessons from this week: (1) keep green-light food handy; and (2) the weight goes back on a whole lot easier than it comes off.' – Karen

'This past week has been really good, although I had a couple of functions where I couldn't follow the diet to the tee (I had a couple of alcoholic drinks and chicken strips with fries and ketchup). The next day it was back to the diet. I felt extremely guilty, but my friends and family told me that it's okay to indulge once in awhile, as long as I keep with my diet the rest of the time, which I do.' – Tammy

'I had a little bump on Friday when I went to a wedding that was a Henry VIII feast but still did way better than I would have had I not been thinking about what was going into my mouth.' – Beverley

'Last night, I made a batch of cookies for a co-worker's birthday and was ridiculously hard on myself for eating one cookie. When I changed my perspective, however, I realised that just a few weeks ago, I would've eaten about a dozen of those cookies and then beat myself up for having done so. Plus, eating that cookie made me think about trade-offs: would I rather eat the cookie or go off my plan in some other way, or would I prefer to use a bit of "wiggle room" to enjoy a glass of wine with dinner one night? There again, I can see that my perspective is changing, and that is of utmost importance for me to succeed, in my opinion.' – Nancy

'The pull of a treat when life is stressful, or when you are on vacation or at a celebratory event can be so profound. I have come to learn over years of dieting that if you slip up and make a bad choice, you need to get back on track ASAP as one mistake can quietly transform into a week of mistakes. I think that process of re-establishing your focus must be critical in successful weight loss.' – Bernadette

Several participants said that the hardest part of the day for them was the evening, when they had the most difficulty steering clear of temptation. Some, like Ross, used green-light snacks to help them:

'I have my hardest time after work during prime snacking time, which was a major downfall period previously. I have put two of my snack times in here. I have managed to eat just green-light snacks, but some nights I still have cravings for the bad stuff. I feel like I imagine an alcoholic does on many nights.'

Although most people find that their cravings do diminish after a few weeks on the Gi Diet because of the levelling effects that green-light eating has on one's blood-sugar levels, there will be times when a craving will surface. Here's how to handle the situation:

1. Try to distract yourself with an activity. Call a friend, fold a basket of laundry, take out the garbage or just go for a walk. Sometimes a craving will pass.

2. If you're still having the craving, pinpoint the flavour you want and find a green-light food that has it. For example, if you want something sweet, have some strawberries or apple sauce; if you want something sweet and creamy, try low-fat yoghurt or ice cream with no added sugar; if you want something salty, have a couple of olives or a dill pickle, or some hummus with veggies; if it's chocolate you want, try half of a chocolate-flavoured nutrition bar or a mug of light instant chocolate. There are many green-light versions of the foods we normally reach for when a craving strikes.

3. Sometimes nothing but a piece of chocolate or peanut butter will do. If this is the case, have a small portion and really enjoy it. Eat it slowly and savour the experience. Chalk it up to that 10 per cent leeway you're allowed on the Gi Diet. Just make sure you're staying green-light 90 per cent of the time.

The good news is that as you continue with your green-light eating, you'll find yourself getting better and better at resisting those bad old foods. Have a look at what e-Clinic participants had to say:

'I'm finding the cravings diminishing since working on this diet, and driving by the fast food places is less tempting as well. I'm encouraged that I can take more control over my eating, which is a relief to my wife!' – J

'Except for the one week I was away plus the wedding, the weight is coming off. I keep expecting to get on the scale and see it's all a mistake. How is it possible to lose five pounds in one week? This has never happened in the past! Don't get me wrong, I'm pleased, but it seems like it's too good to be true.' – Lynn

'It doesn't seem like I'm really on a diet (or doing a "lifestyle change") in general. There are still the occasional times when I have a craving for a Hershey chocolate bar. During times like those, there is a yellow-light quick fix. That's when I'll take a small piece of my wife's organic 70-per-cent-cocoa chocolate bar. It is just enough to take away the craving (the bitterness helps), and stay on the green-light track the rest of the time.' – J

Week 4 Weight		Week 4 Waist		Week 4 Hips	

Week 4 Diary

_____

_____

_____

_____

_____

_____

_____

_____

_____

_____

_____

_____

_____

_____

Optional week 4 meal plan

	Breakfast	Snack	Lunch
Mon	Homey Porridge (page 145) with chopped apple	Wholemeal Fruit Scone (page 183)	Open-face lean deli ham sandwich with lettuce, tomato, red pepper and wholegrain mustard and Basic Gi Salad (page 153)
Tue	Mini Breakfast Puffs (page 147)	Fruit yoghurt	Waldorf Chicken and Rice Salad (page 157)
Wed	Homemade Muesli (page 145) with skimmed milk and fruit yoghurt	Wholemeal Fruit Scone (page 183)	Cottage cheese with apple and grapes, and Basic Gi Salad (page 153)
Thu	Homey Porridge (page 145) with blueberries	Small apple and a glass of skimmed milk	Minestrone Soup (page 150) and Basic Gi Salad (page 153)
Fri	All-Bran with skimmed milk, peach slices and sliced almonds	Fruit yoghurt	½ wholemeal pitta with deli turkey, lettuce, tomato and cucumber, and Basic Gi Salad (page 153)
Sat	Back Bacon Omelette (page 148)	½ food bar	Crab Salad in Tomato Shells (page 158)
Sun	Cinnamon French Toast (page 146) with back bacon	Orange and almonds	Ham and Lentil Soup (page 152) and Basic Gi Salad (page 153)

Week 4 shopping list for meal plan

Produce
Alfalfa sprouts (optional)
Almonds (whole and sliced)
Apples
Asparagus
Aubergines
Baby spinach
Blueberries or mixed summer berries (fresh or frozen)
Broccoli
Carrots
Celery
Cucumbers
Dried apricots
Fresh herbs (basil, chives, coriander, flat-leaf parsley, mint, tarragon)
Garlic

Grapes
Green beans
Lemons
Lettuce (leaf)
Limes
Mushrooms
Onions (yellow and red)
Oranges
Peaches (fresh or canned in juice or water)
Pecans
Peppers (red and green)
Potatoes (new, small)
Spring onions
Strawberries
Sunflower seeds, shelled and unsalted

Snack	Dinner	Snack
Laughing Cow Light cheese with high-fibre crispbread	Salmon Pasta (page 165)	Mixed berries tossed in lime juice with soured cream
Hummus with carrot and celery sticks	Pan-Seared White Fish with Mandarin Salsa (page 169), broccoli and basmati rice	Orange and almonds
Crunchy Chickpeas (page 181)	Chicken Schnitzel (page 171), green beans, carrots and new potatoes	Slice of Strawberry Tea Bread (page 184) and a glass of skimmed milk
Fruit yoghurt	Mushroom and Gravy Pork Chops (page 179), asparagus and basmati rice	½ food bar
Laughing Cow Light cheese with high-fibre crispbread	Horseradish Burgers (page 176) and Tabbouleh Salad (page 156)	Mixed berries tossed in lime juice with soured cream
Hummus with carrot and celery sticks	Vegetarian Moussaka (page 164) and basmati rice	Slice of Strawberry Tea Bread (page 184) and a glass of skimmed milk
Fruit yoghurt	Spicy Roasted Chicken with Tomatoes and Tarragon (page 174), green beans and basmati rice	Slice of One-Bowl Chocolate Cake (page 188) with berries

Tomatoes (large beefsteak, plum, and cherry or grape)
Tomatoes (sun-dried)
Walnuts

Deli
Feta cheese (light)
Hummus (light)
Lean deli ham
Lean deli turkey
Light herb and garlic cream cheese
Parmesan cheese, grated

Bakery
100% stone-ground wholemeal bread
High-fibre crispbread
Wholemeal breadcrumbs
Wholemeal hamburger buns

Wholemeal pitta bread

Fish
Frozen crab
Salmon fillet
White fish fillets

Meat
Back bacon
Beef mince (extra-lean)
Boneless pork loin chops
Chicken breasts (boneless, skinless)

Beans (legumes) and canned vegetables
Chickpeas
Kidney beans (red)
Lentils
Tomatoes (diced)

Tomatoes (plum)
Tomato puree

Pasta and sauces
Macaroni (wholemeal)
Small-shaped pasta (e.g. ditali or tubetti)

Soup and tinned seafood and meat
Chicken stock (low fat, low salt)

Grains and side dishes
Basmati rice
Bulgur wheat

International foods
Rice vinegar

Cooking oil, vinegar, salad dressings and pickles
Buttermilk salad dressing (low fat, low sugar)
Cooking oil spray (vegetable or olive oil)
Dijon mustard
Horseradish
Mayonnaise (fat-free)
Oil (vegetable and extra-virgin olive)
Red wine vinegar
Steak sauce
Wholegrain mustard
Worcestershire sauce

Snacks
Apple sauce (unsweetened)
Food bars (e.g. Slim-Fast)
Tinned mandarin oranges (no added sugar)

Baking
Baking powder
Bicarbonate of soda
Oat bran
Spices (ground allspice, dried basil, black pepper, cayenne pepper, ground cinnamon, ground cumin, Italian herb seasoning, ground nutmeg, oregano, red-pepper flakes, salt, dried thyme)
Splenda
Unsweetened cocoa powder
Vanilla extract
Wheat bran
Wheat germ
Wholemeal flour

Breakfast foods
All-Bran cereal
Oatmeal (large-flake oats)

Beverages
Apple juice (unsweetened)
Dry white wine (or vermouth)

Dairy
Buttermilk
Cottage cheese (low fat)
Fruit yoghurt (non-fat with sweetener)
Laughing Cow cheese (light)
Margarine (soft, non-hydrogenated, light)
Milk (skimmed)
Orange juice (unsweetened)
Soured cream (low fat)

Frozen foods
Mixed berries
Peas (or fresh)

Week 5 Eating Out

It's high time we dealt with the tricky issue of eating out. I say tricky, because unlike when you eat at home, in restaurants you have little control over what goes into the meals and how they are prepared. Nevertheless, there are ways that you can minimise any potential damage.

In restaurants, be especially aware of portion size. Over the past twenty years or so, there has been a dramatic increase in serving sizes – a phenomenon termed 'portion distortion'. Let me give you some examples from a list prepared by the US National Heart, Lung and Blood Institute (see below).

SNACKS	TWENTY YEARS AGO		TODAY	
	size	Calories	size	Calories
Bagel	7.5cm	140	15cm	350
French fries	68g	210	198g	610
Muffin	43g	210	142g	500
Cookie	4cm	55	10cm	275
MEALS		Calories		Calories
Spaghetti and meatballs		500		1025
Turkey sandwich		320		820
Chicken Caesar salad		390		700
Chicken stir-fry		435		865

As you can see, the size and corresponding calories of food have doubled or even tripled over a relatively short period. And we have come to accept these new super-sized portions as standard. A study done with college students on their consumption of their favourite food – macaroni and cheese – shows that the more that was put in front of them, the more they ate. Yet they reported that they felt no fuller on the larger portions than on the smaller ones. Moral: if it's not on your plate, you won't miss it.

While these new super-sizes may look like terrific value, just think what it has cost us in terms of extra pounds and poorer health. Difficult though it may be to refrain from eating everything that has been placed in front of you – I certainly suffer from this – moderation and common sense are your waistline's best friends. Don't feel guilty about leaving food on your plate! In addition to this fundamental recommendation, here are my top ten tips for dining out with family and friends the green-light way.

Top Ten Dining-Out Tips

1. Just before you go out, have a small bowl of high-fibre, green-light cold cereal (such as All-Bran) with skimmed milk and sweetener. I often add a couple of spoonfuls of no-fat/no-sugar fruit yoghurt. This will take the edge off your appetite and get some fibre into your digestive system, which will help reduce the Gi of your upcoming meal.

2. Once seated in the restaurant, drink a glass of water. It will help you feel fuller.

3. Remember to eat slowly to allow your brain the time it needs to realise you're full. Put your fork down between mouthfuls and savour your meal.

4. Once the basket of rolls or bread – which you will ignore! – has been passed round the table, ask the server to remove it. The longer it sits there, the more tempted you will be to dig in.

5. Order a soup or salad first and tell the server you would like this as soon as possible. This will keep you from sitting there hungry while others are filling up on the bread. For soups, go for vegetable- or bean-based, the chunkier the better. Avoid any that are cream-based, such as vichyssoise. For salads, the golden rule is to keep the dressing on the side. Then you can use a fraction of what the restaurant would normally pour over the greens. Avoid Caesar salads, which come pre-dressed and often pack as many calories as a burger.

6. Since you probably won't get boiled new potatoes and can't be sure of what type of rice is being served, ask for double vegetables instead. I have yet to find a restaurant that won't oblige.

7. Stick with low-fat cuts of meat or poultry. If necessary, you can remove the skin. Duck is usually too high in fat. Fish and shellfish are excellent choices but shouldn't be breaded or battered. Tempura is more fat and flour than filling. Remember that servings tend to be generous in restaurants, so eat only 110–170g (4–6oz; the size of a pack of cards) and leave the rest.

8. As with salads, ask for any sauces to be served on the side.

9. For dessert, fresh fruit and berries – without the ice cream – are your best choice. Most other desserts are a dietary disaster. My advice is to avoid dessert. If a birthday cake is being passed around, share your piece with someone. A couple of forkfuls or so along with your coffee should get you off the hook, with minimal dietary damage!

10. Order only decaffeinated coffee. Skimmed-milk decaf cappuccino is our family's favourite choice.

Fast Food

Not so long ago, the idea of getting a green-light lunch at a fast-food outlet was simply laughable. Now, however, partly due to the threat of legal action and a stagnant market share, the major fast-food chains are finally offering some healthy options. Subway has been pioneering the move towards healthy choices for some time, and its initiative has been reflected in its successful growth.

Although things are changing, fast food is still a minefield. Hamburgers are soaked in saturated fat, as are deep-fried chicken and fish. Fries, ketchup, shakes and regular soft drinks are loaded with fat and sugar.

Below, I've listed other good choices in fast food. An asterisk indicates items that are excessively high in sodium – the fast-food industry frequently boosts salt content when lowering fat to make up for any perceived loss of flavour – which can be hazardous to your health.

McDonald's

Salads
Grilled Chicken Caesar Salad (but hold the croutons)

Dressings
Low Fat Newman's Own Balsamic Dressing *

Burgers and sandwiches
Toasted Deli Ham or Chicken Salad (no cheese)

Snack
Fruit Bag

Burger King

Salads
LA Warm Flame-grilled Chicken Salad
LA Warm Crispy Chicken Salad

Dressings
Honey and Mustard
Tomato and Basil

Baguettes
Piri Piri Chicken Baguette

Subway

Note: Best choice of roll is Italian or Wheat.

6-inch Sandwiches with 6g of fat or less

Roast Beef*
Chicken Breast
Ham*
Turkey Breast*
Turkey Breast & Ham*
Sweet Onion Chicken Teriyaki*
Veggie Delite

Deli-Style Sandwiches/Wraps

Ham
Roast Beef
Turkey Breast
Turkey Breast Wrap

Salads
Veggie Delite (side salad)
Grilled Chicken

Dressings
Fat-Free Honey Mustard
Fat-Free Sweet Onion

Note: This information was correct at time of publication. However, as this is a fast-changing marketplace, you may wish to check these restaurants' menus or websites to see if they have expanded their green-light offerings.

On the Road

Being away from home was a challenge for many in the e-Clinic. It is essential to plan ahead when travelling. When I am on the road during media tours, I frequently find myself in situations where there is no green-light food in sight. And these days on planes there is often no food at all. I always carry emergency green-light reserves with me, such as nuts, nutrition bars (usually Slim-Fast), homemade green-light muffins, and fruit.

Breakfast tends to be the biggest challenge of the day because I habitually eat breakfast where I'm staying, as most people do. (For lunch and dinner, there is usually a wider choice of venue and menu.) Fortunately, oatmeal appears to be increasingly available in hotels. Failing that, look for high-fibre cereals, yoghurt and fruit. Skimmed milk is normally available on request. As a last resort, I always carry a couple of pouches of instant oatmeal with me, which requires only the addition of hot water. Though this option is not as good as large-flake oatmeal, it's certainly better than Coco Pops!

If you can get to grips with snacks and breakfast, then staying green-light while travelling is definitely doable.

Here's how e-Clinic participants managed to stay in the green while eating out:

'My toughest struggle this week was stadium food. I went to a football match. You really are at their mercy; they even check handbags on the way in (they say for security, but you aren't even allowed to bring in your own bottle of water). I had no problem skipping the beer, although usually over the course of the match I would have had two or three. The real problem was not so much craving bad food as the unavailability of anything the least bit healthy. I ended up getting a chicken burrito, begging a fork off another vendor, unwrapping the tortilla and eating the chicken, beans, tomatoes and some of the rice. You would think with all the media focus on obesity and healthy eating, someone would open up a salad bar or at least do grilled (as opposed to fried) chicken sandwiches. Maybe there's an opportunity for my second career.' – Karen

'My experience eating regular food at the retreat was really good. I took small amounts of some of the food and left bread and desserts alone. I had cheese sticks, almonds and apples to eat in between meals, which kept me from being as hungry at meal time. I allowed myself one treat: homemade cinnamon rolls. I was really surprised when I came home and had lost weight!' – Diane

'Eating out is still the biggest challenge. I went to a birthday party at East Side Mario's. It is almost impossible to find green-light food there, except for the salad, which I ate generously (dressing on the side and only a little used).' – Lynn

'I was away for four days last week for meetings and training. Because of time constraints it was decided that we would start early in the morning and work as long as possible. The decision was also made to eat breakfast and lunch at the training centre. I arrived the first morning thinking surely there would be something there I could eat. Wrong! What they considered breakfast consisted of giant muffins and croissants, tea and coffee – there weren't even any jugs of water. Lunch was a huge tray of sandwiches (all on white buns or croissants) and a few carrot sticks. There was a big salad with the dressing already tossed in. Although it was some kind of oil and vinegar dressing it was sooo sweet. We were on our own for dinner.

'I decided I needed to take control over the meals I could. When I returned to the hotel I requested a small fridge be delivered to my room. I then went to the grocery store where I bought Fibre 1 cereal, skimmed milk, fruit and disposable bowls, cutlery and bottled water. The next morning I had my breakfast before heading out and felt so much better for it.

When I arrived at the training centre I spoke with the girl responsible for organizing and asked her to direct me to the person preparing our lunches. I spoke to the nicest 'little' lady from the cafeteria and explained that I can't eat sandwiches laden with butter and mayonnaise, and that I needed a salad not all dressed. She was more than happy to oblige. That afternoon, along with all the sandwiches was a plate of cold meat (not non fat but okay), cut up veggies, a half of a boiled egg and a big pickle. There was salad with nothing on it and a small container of oil and vinegar with no sugar added. I was happy.

I will admit that I did have a cocktail after work when everyone met before dinner but I limited myself to one. I know first-hand that alcohol dismisses willpower. I ate dinner out with the group but was as careful as I could be. This allowed me to go to bed without feeling guilty over what I ate that day. I did this for the rest of my stay.

Overall, I know there were things I ate that weren't green-light, but I feel really good about how I handled things. Prior to this I would never have said a word and just ate what was provided for me just so I wouldn't bring attention to myself. But now I realise I am the only one who can control what I eat; I am responsible for myself. I wasn't the least bit embarrassed and no one said a word about my special requests. It was really no big deal after all. Best of all, I feel in control and that feels so good.' – Beverley

Wow, that's tremendous, Beverley! Good luck everyone taking control of your meals while away from home!

| Week 5 Weight | ⬜ | Week 5 Waist | ⬜ | Week 5 Hips | ⬜ |

Week 5 Diary

_____

_____

_____

_____

_____

_____

_____

_____

_____

Optional week 5 meal plan

	Breakfast	Snack	Lunch
Mon	Homey Porridge (page 145) with chopped apple	Cranberry Cinnamon Bran Muffin (page 181)	Open-face chicken sandwich with lettuce, tomato and onion, and Basic Gi Salad (page 153)
Tue	Mini Breakfast Puffs (page 147)	Fruit yoghurt	Gi Pasta Salad (page 156)
Wed	Homemade Muesli (page 145) with skimmed milk and fruit yoghurt	Cranberry Cinnamon Bran Muffin (page 181)	1/2 wholemeal pitta with canned light tuna, lettuce, tomato and cucumber, and Basic Gi Salad (page 153)
Thu	Homey Porridge (page 145) with blueberries	Small apple and a glass of skimmed milk	Quick and Easy Chicken Noodle Soup (page 151) and Basic Gi Salad (page 153)
Fri	All-Bran with skimmed milk, peach slices and sliced almonds	Fruit yoghurt	Mixed Bean Salad (page 157)
Sat	Western Omelette (page 149)	1/2 food bar	Greek Salad (page 155)
Sun	Oatmeal Buttermilk Pancakes with Strawberries (page 146)	Orange and almonds	Tuscan White Bean Soup (page 151) and Basic Gi Salad (page 153)

Snack	Dinner	Snack
Laughing Cow Light cheese with high-fibre crispbread	Easy-Bake Lasagne (page 163) and Caesar Salad (page 166)	Mixed berries tossed in lime juice with soured cream
Hummus with carrot and celery sticks	Gi Fish Fillet (page 166), asparagus carrots and new potatoes	Orange and almonds
Babybel Gouda Lite cheese with crispbread	Chicken Curry (page 170) and Raita Salad (page 152)	Apple Pie Cookie (page 188) and a glass of skimmed milk
Crunchy Chickpeas (page 181)	Vegetable Crumble (page 161) and Tabbouleh Salad page 156)	½ food bar
Laughing Cow Light cheese with high-fibre crispbread	Chicken Fried Rice (page 170)	Mixed berries tossed in lime juice with soured cream
Hummus with carrot and celery sticks	Beef and Aubergine Chilli (page 176) and Basic Gi Salad (page 153)	Apple Pie Cookie (page 188) and a glass of skimmed milk
Babybel Gouda Lite cheese with crispbread	Pork Medallions Dijon (page 178), green beans, carrots and new potatoes	Piece of Plum Crumble (page 186)

Week 5 shopping list for meal plan

Produce
Almonds (whole and sliced)
Apples
Asparagus
Aubergines
Baby spinach
Bean sprouts
Blueberries or mixed summer berries
(fresh or frozen)
Broccoli
Carrots
Celery
Courgettes
Cranberries (dried)
Cucumbers
Fresh herbs (chives, mint, flat-leaf
parsley, sage, tarragon, thyme)
Garlic
Green beans
Kale
Leeks
Lemons
Lettuce (iceberg, leaf and Cos)
Mixed nuts
Mushrooms
Onions (yellow and red)
Oranges
Peaches (fresh or canned in juice or
water)
Peppers (red and green)
Potatoes (new, small)
Plums
Raisins
Sesame seeds
Spring onions
Strawberries
Sunflower seeds (shelled, unsalted)
Sweet potato
Tofu (firm)
Tomatoes (plum)

Deli
Feta cheese (light)
Hummus (light)
Kalamata olives
Parmesan cheese, grated

Bakery
High-fibre crispbread
100% stone-ground wholemeal
bread
Wholemeal pitta bread

Fish
Fish fillets (salmon or trout)

Meat
Back bacon
Beef mince (extra-lean)
Chicken breasts (boneless, skinless)
Pork tenderloins

Beans (legumes) and tinned vegetables
Chickpeas
Kidney beans (red and white)
Mixed beans
Tomatoes (diced)
Tomatoes (plum)
Tomato puree

Pasta and sauces
Lasagne (wholemeal)
Rotini or penne (wholemeal)
Small-shaped pasta (e.g. ditali or
tubetti)
Light tomato sauce (no added sugar)
Low-fat pasta sauce (no cheese or
meat in sauce)

Soup and canned seafood and meat
Anchovy fillets
Chicken stock (low fat, low salt)
Tuna (in water)
Vegetable stock (low fat, low salt)

Grains and side dishes
Basmati rice
Brown rice
Bulgur wheat
Flaxseeds (ground)

International foods
Sesame oil
Soy sauce (low sodium)
Tahini

Cooking oil, vinegar, salad dressings and pickles
Dijon mustard
Cooking oil spray (vegetable or olive oil)
Mayonnaise (fat-free)
Oil (vegetable and extra-virgin olive)
Red wine vinegar
Worcestershire sauce

Snacks
Apple sauce (unsweetened)
Food bars (e.g. Slim-Fast)

Baking
Baking powder
Bicarbonate of soda
Cornflour
Oat bran

Spices (ground cardamom, cayenne pepper, chilli powder, ground cinnamon, ground cumin, curry powder, ground ginger, ground nutmeg, dried oregano, black pepper, red-pepper flakes, salt, dried thyme)
Splenda
Vanilla extract
Wheat bran
Wheat germ
Wholemeal flour

Breakfast foods
All-Bran cereal
Oatmeal (large-flake oats)

Beverages
White wine

Dairy
Buttermilk
Cheddar cheese (low fat)
Cottage cheese (low fat)
Fruit yoghurt (non-fat with sweetener)
Laughing Cow cheese (Light)
Margarine (soft, non-hydrogenated, light)
Milk (skimmed)
Mozzarella cheese (low fat)
Plain yoghurt (non-fat)
Soured cream (light)
Whole Omega-3 eggs

Frozen foods
Mixed berries
Peas (or fresh)

Week 6 Unrealistic Expectations

This week I want to address the critical issue of unrealistic expectations. Unfortunately, in this instant-gratification society, we tend to want immediate results. Even though it took us years to gain the weight we currently have, we expect to lose it extremely quickly. But you can't address a long-term problem like being overweight with a short-term solution. Going to extremes by skipping snacks and cutting calories to a dangerously low level just won't work. Slow, steady weight loss is the only healthy and clinically proven way to lose weight permanently. This is why you need a weight-loss plan you can live with for the long haul, which is what the Gi Diet is all about. One pound a week is the average that most people lose, and it is certainly nothing to sniff at – have you ever seen a pound of fat? It's a substantial amount! And yet look at some of the comments I received from e-Clinic participants:

'Disappointed with my week of "progress." I stuck to the programme pretty good, I even cut back on bread when I wasn't losing at the first of the week. Still only lost one pound.' – Diane

'Feeling disappointed at the small weight loss this week and the little or no change in measurements. I have gone over my meals for the past week to see if there is something I might have done better.' – Kathy (who lost two pounds in one week)

'Small weight loss ... I'll need to get some exercise to start burning off more weight.' – Ross (who lost three pounds in one week)

'Thought maybe I would have lost a little more weight but patience has never been a virtue for me ... ' – another Kathy (who lost four pounds in one week)

All of these people should be feeling happy about their weight loss and proud of their achievements. How unfortunate that they can't give themselves the pat on the back that they so well deserve! Impatience and disappointment in weight-loss success is dangerous: it can derail you from the healthy track you're on and make you want to give up. Just read the following letter from Pat:

'I am really disappointed with myself, as I have only lost one pound this week. I really want the weight to come off faster than it is … I have to tell you, this past Wednesday, mid-afternoon, I started thinking that I was going to pack this programme in. I was thinking again about how the weight wasn't coming off fast enough. But I stopped myself, and asked myself, what really is going on here? Was I hungry, tired or thirsty? I came to the revelation that I was tired and really thirsty. Once I stopped and took a rest and had something to drink, I got refocused. I knew in my heart that quitting wasn't what I wanted to do.'

People often fail on diets because they have unrealistic weight-loss expectations and become impatient. It's great that Pat was able to refocus and stick with the programme. She had been losing an average of over one pound per week, and at that rate she would be reaching her target weight in only nine months. In less than a year she could be at her ideal weight, wearing the clothes she wanted and enjoying her renewed energy and improved health! When you consider the number of years it took to put on the weight, nine months is certainly not an unreasonable timeframe. You know that you are eating in a healthy and nutritious way that is benefiting your body while you reduce. One pound per week is right on target. Yes, there are instances where people have lost three to four pounds per week, but they then frequently hit a plateau and their weight loss averages out to a more normal level. It all depends upon your metabolism, the amount of weight you have to lose and the degree to which you stick to the green-light way of eating.

Here's what can happen if you lose too much too fast:

'This last week I am very impressed with my weight loss, but I have been feeling really foggy. I have vertigo and it has been a very bad week for it. I had to leave work early on Friday due to dizziness. I still feel really foggy today. Do you think that it is due to the diet?' – Tammy

Tammy had been losing an average of three pounds per week for six weeks, and I was concerned that she was overdoing things. I suggested she check that her portion sizes were in line with my recommendations and that she was eating her regular three meals and three snacks per day. I also asked her to see her doctor in case there was some other health issue that needed to be addressed.

To end on a positive note, here's a note I received from Jenny:

'One pound a week for me is really good compared to what I was doing on Weight Watchers (which was about 0.2 pounds a week – very frustrating!).'

Week 6 Weight [ ]	Week 6 Waist [ ]	Week 6 Hips [ ]

Week 6 Diary

_____

_____

_____

_____

_____

_____

_____

_____

Optional week 6 meal plan

	Breakfast	Snack	Lunch
Mon	Homey Porridge (page 145) with chopped apple	Carrot Muffin (page 182)	Open-face lean deli ham sandwich with lettuce, tomato, red pepper and wholegrain mustard, and Basic Gi Salad (page 153)
Tue	Mini Breakfast Puffs (page 147)	Fruit yoghurt	Waldorf Chicken and Rice Salad (page 157)
Wed	Homemade Muesli (page 145) with skimmed milk and fruit yoghurt	Carrot Muffin (page 182)	Cottage cheese with apple and grapes, and Basic Gi Salad (page 153)
Thu	Homey Porridge (page 145) with berries	Small apple and a glass of skimmed milk	Minestrone Soup (page 150) and Basic Gi Salad (page 153)
Fri	All-Bran with skimmed milk, peach slices and sliced almonds	Fruit yoghurt	½ wholemeal pitta with deli turkey, lettuce, tomato and cucumber, and Basic Gi Salad (page 153)
Sat	Italian Omelette (page 148) or Homey Porridge	½ food bar	Crab Salad in Tomato Shells (page 158)
Sun	Cinnamon French Toast (page 146) with back bacon	Orange and almonds	Ham and Lentil Soup (page 152) and Basic Gi Salad (page 153)

Snack	Dinner	Snack
Laughing Cow Light cheese with high-fibre crispbread	Fettuccine Primavera (page 159) and Caesar Salad (page 154)	Mixed berries tossed in lime juice with soured cream
Hummus with carrot and celery sticks	Ginger Wasabi Halibut (page 167), Cold Noodle Salad with Cucumber and Sesame (page 155), snow peas and carrots	Orange and almonds
Cottage cheese (low fat) with peach slices	Chicken Tarragon with Mushrooms (page 173), broccoli and basmati rice	Pecan Brownie (page 189) and a glass of skimmed milk
Crunchy Chickpeas (page 181)	Meatloaf (page 175), green beans, carrots and new potatoes	½ food bar
Laughing Cow Light cheese with high-fibre crispbread	Bean and Onion Pizza (page 162)	Mixed berries tossed in lime juice with soured cream
Hummus with carrot and celery sticks	Grilled Tuna with Chimichurri Sauce (page 168), asparagus and new potatoes	Pecan Brownie (page 189) and a glass of skimmed milk
Fruit yoghurt	Orange Chicken with Almonds (page 172), green beans and basmati rice	Slice of Apple Raspberry Coffee Cake (page 187)

Week 6 shopping list for meal plan

Produce
Almonds (whole and sliced)
Apples
Asparagus
Baby spinach
Blueberries or mixed summer berries
(fresh or frozen)
Broccoli
Carrots
Celery
Courgettes (yellow)
Cucumbers
Fresh herbs (basil, chives, coriander,
flat-leaf parsley)
Garlic
Ginger root
Grapes
Green beans
Lemon
Lettuce (leaf and Cos)
Limes
Mangetout
Mushrooms
Onions (yellow and red)
Oranges
Peaches (fresh or canned in juice or
water)
Pecans
Peppers (red and green)
Potatoes (new, small)
Raisins
Raspberries
Sesame seeds
Spring onions
Strawberries
Sunflower seeds, shelled and
unsalted
Tofu (firm)
Tomatoes (large beefsteak and plum)
Tomatoes (sun-dried)
Walnuts

Deli
Feta cheese (light)
Hummus (light)
Lean deli ham
Lean deli turkey
Parmesan cheese, grated

Bakery
High-fibre crispbread
100% stone-ground wholemeal
bread
Wholemeal pitta bread

Fish
Frozen crab
Halibut fillets
Tuna steaks (1/2-inch thick)

Meat
Back bacon
Beef mince (extra-lean)
Chicken breasts (boneless, skinless)

Beans (legumes) and canned vegetables
Chickpeas
Kidney beans (red and white)
Lentils
Tomatoes (plum)
Tomato purée

Pasta and sauces
Capellini or spaghetti (wholemeal)
Fettuccine or linguine (wholemeal)
Low-fat pasta sauce (no cheese or
meat in sauce)
Small-shaped pasta (ditali or tubetti)

Soup and tinned seafood and meat
Anchovy fillets
Chicken stock (low fat, low salt)
Vegetable stock (low fat, low salt)

Grains and side dishes
Basmati rice
Flaxseeds (ground)

International foods
Mirin (or sweet sherry)
Rice vinegar
Sesame seeds (toasted)
Soy sauce (low salt)
Tahini
Wasabi powder

Cooking oil, vinegar, salad dressings and pickles
Buttermilk salad dressing (low fat, low sugar)
Cooking oil spray (vegetable or olive oil)
Dijon mustard
Oil (vegetable and extra-virgin olive)
Red wine vinegar
Wholegrain mustard
Worcestershire sauce

Snacks
Food bars (e.g. Slim-Fast)

Baking
Active dry yeast
Baking powder
Bicarbonate of Soda
Brown-sugar substitute
Cornflour
Oat bran
Spices (black pepper, cayenne pepper, cinnamon, ground ginger, ground nutmeg, dried oregano, red-pepper flakes, salt, dried tarragon, dried thyme)

Splenda
Unsweetened cocoa powder
Vanilla extract
Wheat bran
Wheat germ
Wholemeal flour

Breakfast foods
All-Bran cereal
Oatmeal (large-flake oats)

Beverages
Tomato juice
Vegetable cocktail juice
Vermouth or white wine

Dairy
Buttermilk
Cottage cheese (low fat)
Fruit yoghurt (non-fat with sweetener)
Laughing Cow cheese (Light)
Margarine (soft, non-hydrogenated, light)
Milk (skimmed)
Mozzarella cheese (low fat)
Soured cream (low fat)
Whole Omega-3 eggs

Frozen food
Peas (or fresh)
Mixed berries

Week 7 Emotional Eating

This week we cover the whole question of emotional eating, frequently described as using 'food for comfort'. I have asked my wife, Dr Ruth Gallop, who is Professor Emeritus at the University of Toronto, to write this section, as one of her specialties is childhood trauma and how that plays out in adult life. This has given her considerable insight into the role food plays in helping people deal with their emotional issues. We realise that this is a very large topic but hope to provide you with some guidance. Here are her thoughts.

We all eat for comfort to a lesser or greater extent. When we are sick many of us have favourite foods – often foods from our childhood that we associate with being looked after. There are foods we eat rarely and foods we could eat every day – often foods that make us feel good or satiated.

When we have reasonably balanced lives, food plays an important but not dominant role in our day-to-day lives. When our lives are out of balance and we don't feel good about certain aspects of them, then food can take over. When we don't feel good about ourselves, food can be a powerful and damaging force. This is particularly true for women because our society is fixated on how we should look. Putting aside all the health reasons for being at a 'normal' weight, our society just doesn't approve of fat people. And more importantly fat people often don't approve of themselves.

Eating to feel better is usually preceded by negative feelings. For some people, these feelings may include sadness, loneliness or even a sense of boredom. For others, the feelings can be more in the range of anger, irritability or high stress. These feelings can lead to a vicious eating cycle. It goes something like this:

I feel angry/bored/sad/bad about myself (low self-esteem) ➜ *so I eat to feel better* ➜ *I experience a brief blood sugar high and feel better* ➜ *I experience a blood sugar crash and feel terrible* ➜ *I feel bad about myself for eating, for failing* ➜ *so I eat to feel better ... and around I go.*

In many situations the original reasons for feeling bad about oneself or getting angry, overwhelmed or disappointed, may have origins in childhood, but overeating, negative body image and low self-esteem are the present consequences. We do not make any conscious link between past events and current behaviour. For example, parental approval and love may have been connected with food via treats or eating all that was put in front of us. Or we may have been punished (love withdrawn) if we didn't eat our vegetables. Eating becomes connected with trying to recapture that good feeling of being loved. Although we are unaware of these motives or psychological reasons for the behaviour, we have done it for so long it becomes part of our food and eating habits.

Rick's mother cannot bear to see food left unfinished on the plate, regardless of whether or not a person is still hungry. At ninety-seven years of age, she still says, 'I do like to see a clean plate,' when all the food on the table has disappeared. I have learned to deal with this learned behaviour – a behaviour that earned Rick love and approval from his mother when he was a child – by never putting excess food on the table at mealtimes or putting out bowls of food for individual selection. Otherwise, Rick's impulse will be to finish the food, and he will unconsciously graze.

How do you change eating behaviours that you learned as a child? First, you have taken the most important step by removing all red-light food from the house and making a conscious decision to eat only green-light foods – a huge step! Make sure you reward yourself for this accomplishment. Give yourself a treat (just make sure it isn't a red-light food).

Become conscious of your eating habits. For example, when you walk in the front door, is your first stop the fridge or snack cupboard? When you have had a bad day at work or the kids have been a hassle do you deal with it by eating something sweet or high fat? When you feel bored and have nothing structured to do, is food the first thing you think of? Are you unable to watch TV without snacking, so large amounts of food pass into your mouth without you realizing? I have one piece of dark chocolate most evenings if I am watching TV. The other night I realised I was in the middle of eating a second piece with no memory of reaching down and picking it up!

Take a day or two to jot down your eating patterns, noting when automatic behaviours take over and when it is most difficult for you to avoid eating in excess. You'll soon begin to recognise your 'at-risk' situations. If food comforts you when you're stressed or setting unrealistic expectations for yourself, such as getting all the errands done, cooking all the meals and doing all the child care, you'll start to recognise your patterns and can then start to consider alternative ways to cope, for example, sharing tasks with others.

Some emotional eating habits to watch out for include:

- Grazing. This is a well-established teenage habit that many have not grown out of. If you cannot pass a fridge without opening it, grazing is a habit for you.

- Eating when stressed, angry, irritable, tired or frustrated.

- Eating when sad, bored or lonely.

- Eating too quickly. Never gobble your food. Remember it takes twenty to thirty minutes for the stomach to tell the brain it is full.

- Eating unconsciously. Never eat from large packages of food. Instead, put the small portion you plan to eat in a bowl or on a plate.

- Eating too-large portions. Thanks to fast-food and family restaurants, many portion sizes have doubled in recent years, and we have brought this 'portion distortion' into our homes.

- Always eating during any social activity, such as sports events, visits and having coffee with a friend.

Once you have recognised your own unhealthy eating behaviours, change by modifying one behaviour at a time. For example, if you usually walk in the front door and immediately go to the fridge to get a snack, consider it one of your snack times and ensure that you have a green-light snack ready. If you usually eat while watching television in the evenings, make a list of pleasurable activities you could be doing instead of eating. How about putting together a photo album, knitting or even ironing while watching your favourite shows? Or are there pleasurable things you could do instead of watching TV, like doing a crossword puzzle, going for a walk, taking a class to learn a fun hobby or even having a hot bath? Substituting pleasurable activities helps break the vicious cycle I have described above. To start the process, write out a list below of substitute activities you enjoy.

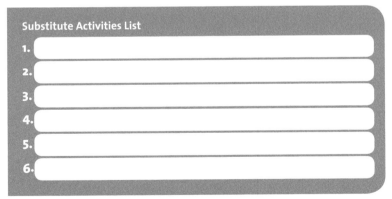

Substitute Activities List
1.
2.
3.
4.
5.
6.

This list will be an important tool to help break those bad eating habits. Use it until you feel sure that your new behaviours and eating patterns are your new habits. And don't beat yourself up if you slip – it happens to all of us. Just get back on the wagon. Having the determination to do this programme deserves a pat on the back, so be sure to reward yourself for your small triumphs – go to a show or game, or buy some flowers or a new CD.

Emotional eating is a subject that resonated with e-Clinic participants, many of whom have struggled with their weight since childhood.

'I had some 'emotional' eating this week. On Tuesday, my doctor told me my X-rays were clear for pneumonia, but there were spots in the lower lungs. That night I had a steak and some red wine. I figured if I had lung cancer I'd lose weight anyway, so what the hell? Had a CT scan on Wednesday and on Friday found out the spots were scars from previous bouts of bronchitis/pneumonia. That led to a celebratory glass of wine (or two) with dinner. I'm back on track now, but this has been a roller-coaster week.' – Karen

'I have gained two pounds this week. Disappointed and angry with myself definitely. I can only say that this is a result of emotional eating this week. My stress level at work was at a high level ... One day mid-week, my commuting friend bought me a large chocolate-covered marshmallow on a stick as she knew that this was a treat my mother and I shared at this time of the year. In addition to this, I have been having a lot of dreams of my deceased parents ... All I can say is lesson learned and now another week begins and I must get back on track because losing the weight is extremely important to me ... I didn't realise until I started this programme how much of an emotional eater I am.' – P

'Your wife's comments on the emotional aspect of eating and food really hit home. I have to constantly work on this. I think we all know we are doing it, but at the time you do it anyway and fuel the cycle. I'm looking at some sort of hobby to turn to instead of the fridge. Or I guess I could take up smoking and drinking instead ... Just kidding!' – Ross

'I've been through a lot in the past few years (a divorce followed by an abusive relationship), and I know I gained all the extra weight in some effort to "protect" myself. I am trying to learn to love myself in ways that do not involve reaching for food as a means of consoling myself. I have a long way to go, but I have the basic tools – plus, I'm on my own now and safe. The stronger I get financially and emotionally, the more I care about my health and appearance.' – Nancy

Keep in mind that as you lose weight you will feel better not only physically but also psychologically. Being successful will improve your self-esteem. Feeling better about how you look is the best reinforcement for holding back on red-light foods, and breaking those bad eating habits. You will notice your body changing and others will too. As you start to experience success in permanent weight reduction you will think of yourself as successful. Successful people hold their bodies differently and interact with people differently. As a reader once said, 'I no longer hide behind a tree every time a camera comes out.' You may find you feel safe enough to come out into the world. Let people compliment you.

Week 7 Diary

_____

_____

_____

_____

_____

_____

_____

_____

_____

_____

_____

Optional week 7 meal plan

	Breakfast	Snack	Lunch
Mon	Homey Porridge (page 145) with chopped apple	Apple Bran Muffin (page 182)	Open-face chicken sandwich with lettuce, tomato and onion, and Basic Gi Salad (page 153)
Tue	Mini Breakfast Puffs (page 147)	Fruit yoghurt	Gi Pasta Salad (page 156)
Wed	Homemade Muesli (page 145) with skimmed milk and fruit yoghurt	Apple Bran Muffin (page 182)	1/2 wholemeal pitta with canned light tuna, lettuce, tomato and cucumber, and Basic Gi Salad (page 153)
Thu	Homey Porridge (page 145) with blueberries	Small apple and a glass of skimmed milk	Quick and Easy Chicken Noodle Soup (page 151) and Basic Gi Salad (page 153)
Fri	All-Bran with skimmed milk, peach slices and sliced almonds	Fruit yoghurt	Mixed Bean Salad (page 157)
Sat	Vegetarian Omelette (page 149) or Homey Porridge (page 145)	1/2 food bar	Greek Salad (page 155)
Sun	Oatmeal Buttermilk Pancakes with Strawberries (page 146)	Orange and almonds	Tuscan White Bean Soup (page 151) and Basic Gi Salad (page 153)

Snack	Dinner	Snack
Laughing Cow Light cheese with high-fibre crispbread	Rigatoni with Mini-Meat Balls (page 177) and Caesar Salad (page 154)	Mixed berries tossed in lime juice with soured cream
Hummus with carrot and celery sticks	Citrus-Poached Haddock (page 167), green beans and new potatoes	Orange and almonds
Fruit yoghurt	Chicken Jambalaya (page 172) and broccoli	Creamy Lemon Square (page 190) and a glass of skimmed milk
Crunchy Chickpeas (page 181)	Barley Risotto with Leeks, Lemon and Peas (page 160) and Tabbouleh Salad (page 158)	½ food bar
Laughing Cow Light cheese with high-fibre crispbread	Thai Red Curry Prawn Pasta (page 166)	Mixed berries tossed in lime juice with soured cream
Hummus with carrot and celery sticks	Zesty Barbecued Chicken (page 174), Tangy Red and Green Coleslaw (page 153) and new potatoes	Creamy Lemon Square (page 190) and a glass of skimmed milk
Yoghurt with peach slices	Pork Tenderloin with Apple Compote (page 180), Brussels sprouts, carrots and new potatoes	Piece of Berry Crumble (page 185)

Week 7 shopping list for meal plan

Produce
Almonds (whole and sliced)
Apples
Aubergines
Blueberries or mixed summer berries (fresh or frozen)
Broccoli
Brussels sprouts
Cabbage (green and red)
Carrots
Celery
Courgettes
Cucumbers
Currants
Fresh herbs (chives, coriander, flat-leaf parsley, mint, rosemary, sage and thyme)
Garlic
Green beans
Kale
Leek
Lemons
Lettuce (leaf, iceberg and Cos)
Limes
Mushrooms
Onions (yellow and red)
Oranges
Peaches (fresh or canned in juice or water)
Pecans
Peppers (red and green)
Potatoes (new, small)
Spring onions
Strawberries
Sunflower seeds, shelled and un-salted
Tomatoes (plum)

Deli
Feta cheese (low fat)
Hummus (light)
Kalamata olives
Parmesan cheese, grated

Bakery
High-fibre crispbread
100% stone-ground wholemeal bread
Wholemeal pitta bread

Fish
Haddock fillets
Shrimp (large raw)

Meat
Chicken breasts (boneless, skinless)
Lean chicken or turkey mince
Pork tenderloin

Beans (legumes) and tinned vegetables
Chickpeas
Kidney beans (red and white)
Mixed beans
Tomatoes (plum)
Tomatoes (stewed)
Tomato puree

Pasta and sauces
Fusilli or penne (wholemeal)
Macaroni or small shells (whole-meal)
Rigatoni (wholemeal)
Spaghetti or linguine (wholemeal)
Small-shaped pasta (e.g. ditali or tubetti)
Light tomato sauce

Soup and tinned seafood and meat
Anchovy fillets
Chicken stock (low fat, low salt)
Tuna (light, in water)
Vegetable stock (low fat, low salt)

Grains and side dishes
Barley
Brown rice
Bulgur wheat
Flaxseeds (ground)

International foods
Tahini
Thai red curry paste

Cooking oil, vinegar, salad dressings and pickles
Cider vinegar
Cooking oil spray (vegetable or olive oil)
Dijon mustard
Mayonnaise (fat free)
Oil (vegetable and extra-virgin olive)
Red wine vinegar
Worcestershire sauce

Snacks
Apple sauce (unsweetened)
Food bars (e.g. Slim-Fast)

Baking
Baking powder
Bicarbonate of soda
Brown-sugar substitute
Cornflour
Ground almonds
Oat bran
Spices (ground allspice, bay leaves, black pepper, cayenne pepper, celery seeds, chilli powder, ground cinnamon, ground cloves, ground cumin, dried oregano, dried sage, salt and dried thyme)

Splenda
Vanilla extract
Wheat bran
Wheat germ
Wholemeal flour

Breakfast foods
All-Bran cereal
Oatmeal (large-flake oats)

Beverages
Apple juice (unsweetened)
Dry white wine (or vermouth)

Dairy
Buttermilk
Cheddar cheese (low fat)
Fruit yoghurt (non-fat with sweetener)
Laughing Cow cheese (light)
Margarine (soft, non-hydrogenated, light)
Milk (skimmed)
Orange juice (unsweetened)
Soured cream (low fat)
Whole omega-3 eggs

Frozen foods
Frozen apple-juice concentrate
Mixed berries
Peas (or fresh)

Week 8 Reaching a Plateau

When you're rigorously adhering to the green-light way and have been steadily losing weight for many successive weeks, it's difficult to accept that the weight loss should suddenly stall. Unfair as it may be, it is inevitable. Weight loss never occurs in a straight line, but always in a series of steps or plateaus, as all of our e-Clinic participants discovered at one point or another:

'I am totally surprised and very disappointed. This week I made sure that I ate only green knowing that I had two dinners out for my birthday. I even went online and checked the menus at both places so I could go in knowing exactly what I was going to have and not be tempted by everything else. I skipped the bread basket, the desserts, had grilled chicken and salad with vinaigrette dressing at one place, and grilled salmon, fresh beans and baby carrots, and salad with vinaigrette dressing on my birthday. The only thing I did have was a small glass of wine. No cake, didn't eat one of my favourite cookies fresh from Tim Horton's that were bought by one of the girls I ride in with on the bus, since we couldn't have a cake, she said. I was so pleased with myself – that was until I stepped on the scale this morning and it showed the 1.5 pound gain and no change in measurements. I just don't understand. I'm at a loss, frustrated and very disappointed.' – Kathy

'Battling a tough weekly result. I'm a little baffled at my lack of weight loss this week, and due to the results I had a bout of emotional eating with a box of Timbits. I find it really frustrating (and I've been here before) to do a total 180 on my eating and not have any weight come off.' – Sandra

'Well, I have found a plateau, but since I knew it was out there waiting for me and this is a marathon not a sprint, I'm okay with it – after a few moments of "black cloud." As long as things keep moving forward ... ' – Ross

Many factors show up on the scale: stress, water retention, hormonal shifts, change in exercise schedules, even seasonality. The body tends to naturally want to put on weight for winter and lose a bit for summer due to the feast-and-famine cycles from deep in our ancestral past. Oestrogen levels particularly can influence how much water you retain, which is why women experience sudden short-term changes in weight, particularly before a period – and even more so during menopause. Menopause, which can go on for up to ten years, can impact a woman's weight in two ways. First, oestrogen levels decrease, causing erratic swings in water retention and blood sugar levels. When your blood-sugar levels drop, your brain calls for more sugar, making you want to reach out for those red-light foods, which will temporarily give you a boost and make you feel better in the short term. However, the sugar high will cause your insulin to kick in, quickly bringing your blood-sugar levels down to another low. We know all about this relentless cycle. That's why it's so important to eat only green-light foods, because they will help stabilise your blood sugar and mood.

Second, menopause will slow your metabolic rate, or the rate at which your body burns calories. As you're aware, to lose weight, you have to use up more calories than your body takes in. So if you are burning fewer calories, your rate of weight loss will slow. This is why it can be more of a challenge to lose weight during menopause.

So for many reasons, your weight can fluctuate significantly even day to day. This is why I suggest you restrict your weigh-in to once a week, and why I think it would be better to weigh in only once a month. Then you'd avoid the disappointment of these short-term aberrations and focus on your long-term success. You are playing the averages and must have patience. Just keep on the green-light track and the weight will continue to come off. Some e-Clinic participants also wondered why they sometimes seemed to be losing inches but not pounds, and sometimes pounds but not inches. Remember, everyone is different, and weight loss doesn't ever happen in a straight line; eventually both the inches and pounds will come off – guaranteed!

So don't let an irregularity on the scale get you down. Though nothing is quite as frustrating as hitting a weight-loss plateau, if you hang in there – and don't use food to console yourself – you will reach your weight-loss target. Here is how some e-Clinic participants tried to focus on the positive as they came to terms with their plateaus:

'I thought I had done well this week and was sure I had a good loss ... It was disappointing when the scale said I'd only lost half a pound and virtually nothing in inches. I can't believe that with the amount of weight I have to lose that my body would be considering plateauing yet! I know I feel good and that I made good decisions this week, but I just didn't see any rewards. I don't know if how much my monthly cycle plays in this as I was on all week ... Oh well, as they say, Rome wasn't built in a day and I'm not going to lose all this weight in a day, a month or even a year (sounds daunting!)' – Kathy

'I like to weigh myself daily because I feel it keeps me on track. It does not discourage me. I have always done it that way. The only exception I make is if I know I had a really bad day then I will wait a day to weigh myself. But I have noticed since my weight has been going down that it will be down for a few days then pop back up to the older weight and then a few days later back down it will go. The encouraging part is that each time it goes up it is not as far as the time before.' – Diane

Week 8 Weight	☐	Week 8 Waist	☐	Week 8 Hips	☐

Week 8 Diary

_____

_____

_____

_____

_____

_____

_____

_____

Optional week 8 meal plan

	Breakfast	Snack	Lunch
Mon	Homey Porridge (page 145) with chopped apple	Wholemeal Fruit Scone (page 183)	Open-face lean deli ham sandwich with lettuce, tomato, red pepper and wholegrain mustard, and Basic Gi Salad (page 153)
Tue	Mini Breakfast Puffs (page 147)	Fruit yoghurt	Waldorf Chicken and Rice Salad (page 157)
Wed	Homemade Muesli (page 145) with skimmed milk and fruit yoghurt	Wholemeal Fruit Scone (page 183)	Cottage cheese with apple and grapes, and Basic Gi Salad (page 153)
Thu	Homey Porridge (page 145) with blueberries	Small apple and a glass of skimmed milk	Minestrone Soup (page 150) and Basic Gi Salad (page 153)
Fri	All-Bran with skimmed milk, peach slices and sliced almonds	Fruit salad	½ wholemeal pitta with deli turkey, lettuce, tomato and cucumber, and Basic Gi Salad (page 153)
Sat	Back Bacon Omelette (page 148) or Homey Porridge (page 145)	½ food bar	Crab Salad and Tomato Shells (page 158)
Sun	Cinnamon French Toast (page 146) with back bacon	Orange and almonds	Ham and Lentil Soup (page 152) and Basic Gi Salad (page 153)

Snack	Dinner	Snack
Laughing Cow Light cheese with high-fibre crispbread	Salmon Pasta (page 165)	Mixed berries tossed in lime juice with soured cream
Hummus with carrot and celery sticks	Pan-Seared White Fish with Mandarin Salsa (page 169), broccoli and basmati rice	Orange and almonds
Cottage cheese (low fat) with peach slices	Chicken Schnitzel (page 171), green beans, carrots and new potatoes	Slice of Strawberry Tea Bread (Page 184) and a glass of skimmed milk
Crunchy Chickpeas (page 181)	Mushroom and Gravy Pork Chops (page 179), asparagus and basmati rice	½ food bar
Laughing Cow Light cheese with high-fibre crispbread	Horseradish Burgers (page 176) and Tabbouleh Salad (page 156)	Mixed berries tossed in lime juice with soured cream
Hummus with carrot and celery sticks	Vegetarian Moussaka (page 164) and basmati rice	Slice of Strawberry Tea Bread (page 184) and a glass of skimmed milk
Fruit yoghurt	Spicy Roasted Chicken with Tomatoes and Tarragon (page 174), green beans and basmati rice	Slice of One-Bowl Chocolate Cake (page 188) with berries

Week 8 shopping list for meal plan

Produce
Alfalfa sprouts (optional)
Almonds (whole and sliced)
Apples
Asparagus
Aubergines
Baby spinach
Blueberries or mixed summer berries
(fresh or frozen)
Broccoli
Carrots
Celery
Cucumbers
Dried apricots
Fresh herbs (basil, chives, coriander,
flat-leaf parsley, mint, tarragon)
Garlic
Grapes
Green beans
Lemons
Lettuce (leaf)
Limes
Mushrooms
Onions (yellow and red)
Oranges
Peaches (fresh or canned in juice or
water)
Pecans
Peppers (red and green)
Potatoes (new, small)
Spring onions
Strawberries
Sunflower seeds, shelled and
unsalted
Tomatoes (large beefsteak, plum,
and cherry or grape)
Tomatoes (sun-dried)
Walnuts

Deli
Feta cheese (light)
Hummus (light)
Lean deli ham
Lean deli turkey
Light herb and garlic cream cheese
Parmesan cheese, grated

Bakery
High-fibre crispbread
100% stone-ground wholemeal
bread
Wholemeal breadcrumbs
Wholemeal hamburger buns
Wholemeal pitta bread

Fish
Frozen crab
Salmon fillet
White fish fillets

Meat
Back bacon
Beef mince (extra-lean)
Boneless pork loin chops
Chicken breasts (boneless, skinless)

Beans (legumes) and tinned
vegetables
Chickpeas
Kidney beans (red)
Lentils
Tomatoes (chopped)
Tomatoes (plum)
Tomato puree

Pasta and sauces
Macaroni (wholemeal)
Small-shaped pasta (ditali or tubetti)

Soup and tinned seafood and meat
Chicken stock (low fat, low salt)

Grains and side dishes
Basmati rice
Bulgur

International foods
Rice vinegar

Cooking oil, vinegar, salad dressings and pickles
Buttermilk salad dressing (low fat, low sugar)
Cooking oil spray (vegetable or olive oil)
Dijon mustard
Horseradish
Mayonnaise (fat-free)
Oil (vegetable and extra-virgin olive)
Red wine vinegar
Steak sauce
Wholegrain mustard
Worcestershire sauce

Snacks
Apple sauce (unsweetened)
Canned mandarin oranges (no added sugar)
Food bars (e.g. Slim-Fast)

Baking
Baking powder
Bicarbonate of Soda
Oat bran
Spices (ground allspice, dried basil, black pepper, cayenne pepper, ground cinnamon, ground cumin, Italian herb seasoning, ground nutmeg, oregano, red-pepper flakes, salt, dried thyme)

Splenda
Unsweetened cocoa powder
Vanilla extract
Wheat bran
Wheat germ
Wholemeal flour

Breakfast foods
All-Bran cereal
Oatmeal (large-flake oats)

Beverages
Apple juice (unsweetened)
Dry white wine (or vermouth)

Dairy
Buttermilk
Cottage cheese (low fat)
Fruit yoghurt (non-fat with sweetener)
Laughing Cow cheese (light)
Margarine (soft, non-hydrogenated, light)
Milk (skimmed)
Orange juice (unsweetened)
Soured cream (low fat)

Frozen foods
Mixed berries
Peas (or fresh)

Week 9 Staying Motivated

We are now nearly two-thirds of the way through the first thirteen weeks of the Gi Diet – it's a great time to reflect on your progress to date and what still needs to be done to keep your motivation high. Over the past eight weeks, e-Clinic participants have reported a wide range of results. Some have taken to the green-light way of eating like the proverbial duck to water; while others have struggled to make the transition from their red-light habits. Most of the problems participants experienced had nothing to do with the diet, but with stress, emotions, work and home pressures and non-related health issues. The common thread, however, was that they were all determined to get that weight devil off their backs. This week I want to discuss keeping determination strong. You wouldn't be human if you didn't feel your resolve starting to waver from time to time. When it does, there are a number of things you can do to encourage yourself to keep going:

1. Remember your initial reasons

Reread your reasons for wanting to lose weight on page 41. Remember why it was so important to you to slim down when you started this journey and why you need to persevere.

2. Use physical reminders of your goal

Keep a picture of an outfit you're going to buy when you reach your goal, or a photograph of a thinner you where you will see it every day.

'A picture or two of yourself really helps, I think. Although you know you are overweight, your mental picture of yourself is not of an overweight person. I can only speak for myself here. Once I saw some pictures of how I really looked, how I looked to others, and that was a big help in motivating me.' – Ross

'I am using my beautiful red leather coat to motivate me. Last winter when I went to put it on, it was about two inches too small. I was not able to close the zipper. Now when I put the coat on, I am able to zip it up. Tight yes, but I know that I have made progress. What an incredible feeling ... I am determined to wear the coat this winter.' – P

'I had reached the point where I knew I had to buy clothing in the Big Women's section of a shop. I was determined that was not going to happen again.

I dropped almost two stone, and I know I had reached a comfort level with how my old clothing was fitting. I think to some extent not buying new clothing backfired. With my clothes falling off me, I no longer felt the strain on the waistband, so I overindulged. So, I've done two things: I've gone into the wardrobe and found even smaller clothes than the ones that now fit. I am wearing clothes (not out in public!) that are much too tight. The discomfort is a reminder that I've got a long way to go. And secondly, I recently went shopping for new clothes. Instead of trying on a buying a size 16 (which I am now down to), I found the prettiest things I could find in a 12 and 14, which are not available in my size. I tried them on in the changing room to get an idea of how much more I have to do before I can just walk into a shop and pick up anything I like.' – Karen

3. Keep in mind how far you've come

Compare yourself now to where you were before you started the diet. How much weight have you lost? How much better do your clothes fit you? How has your energy level and health improved? What can you do now that you couldn't do before? Going back to your old eating habits won't seem so tempting when you think how it will undermine all the good things that weight loss has brought you so far.

'I realised this morning that I am no longer experiencing heartburn at night, which is an added bonus.' – Nancy

'I did notice yesterday when I put on a sweatshirt from last year that it was big. What a great feeling. When I was putting away my summer clothes, I said to myself, "I won't be using these again." What a motivator.' – P

'This may sound strange, but I am beginning to notice that everything tastes better, and in turn foods that are very salty are almost unpalatable.' – Bernadette

'I've officially broken below 260, something I've never accomplished before on any other diet. I'm so excited!' – J

'I have so much more energy this season than I did a year ago. I can remember last year I didn't even want to put up my Christmas decorations because I just did not have any energy. This year I feel back to my old self, now I just need to find that self that I haven't seen since around 1995! I know I can do this!' – Diane

4. Try the 'shopping bag cure'

Often, people don't realise how much weight actually weighs. Sounds crazy, but when people tell me they've lost 'only' one and a half stone, I ask them to fill a couple of shopping bags with one and a half stone of books and carry them up and down the stairs a few times. Everyone is always glad to put the bags down and report that they had no idea how heavy one and a half stone really is.

So the next time you're feeling uninspired, fill a shopping bag or two with the amount of books or cans of food that equal how much weight you've lost over the last eight weeks of the programme and carry them up and down a flight of stairs three times. You'll be amazed at what you've lost, and you'll be so relieved to put the bag down. You couldn't have put that weight down weeks ago, when it was still around your waist, hips and thighs!

Keep the bag intact, and add more books or cans as you continue to lose weight. It's a wonderful motivator.

'Many years ago I had lost a lot of weight. When I was at a 20-pound loss, a dear skinny friend said to me, "Diana, do you realise you have lost the equivalent of a 20-pound bag of potatoes? Just carry that around for a while to see how much you have lost." I have often thought about that. And yes, I have noticed a big difference in my energy level; going up and down steps is not nearly as hard. My joints do not ache as much and my blood pressure is so much better. And my clothes are also fitting better. So even though I've lost "only 1 stone", I am feeling the effects and do not want to go backwards!' – Diane

'At last, I'm below the dreaded 21 stone – never to be seen again! ... I didn't think this day would ever arrive. Although one and a half stone doesn't seem like a lot if you look at the whole picture, it was my first target in my journey ... It's one and a half stone in the right direction, and when I held one and a half stone of kitty litter in the store, I realised it's a lot of weight to be carrying every day – no wonder my knees and back hurt!' – Kathy

5. Get support

Buddy up with friends, a spouse or family members who are trying to lose weight. They will give you a sense of camaraderie and encouragement as you strive for your goal, and you can turn to them for support when you need it.

'The best way to stay motivated is to do the programme with someone else. My Gi Jane group has been a fantastic source of inspiration and motivation. When one of us is down, the others pick us up. When we are all down at the same time, we have a group meeting and re-kindle the reasons we are doing all of this.' – Lynn

'My friend Kathy is also part of this programme. Part of our weekly chat is to check with one another on our progress and to provide support. We are good at giving each other praise when it is appropriate and providing words of encouragement too. We also discuss our accomplishments and challenges. It really helps to have a good buddy system. It makes the journey easier.' – Pat

'My kids are young but very supportive, as I have told them I am trying to make better food choices so that I will be healthy for a long time. (They have decided that this means I will be able to baby-sit when I am a grandma to their kids! They are only six and nine!) – Bernadette

'The holiday barrage of social events starts this coming Friday night but I think I have that one under control. I had a long conversation with a male friend and told him what I have been doing, which was a surprise in itself as I don't normally share that kind of information. But he was thrilled and is so supportive – it really felt good. And he will also be at the Friday event.' – Kathy

6. Try the £5 cure

This is a motivator that people often stumble upon by accident. The siren song of a red-light lunch draws them into a fast-food chain where they order a burger with the works, a large serving of French fries and a shake. Mid-afternoon, they feel lousy and can barely keep their eyes open – they've found out the hard way where straying from the green-light path gets you.

'When you mentioned in your book how horrible you'd feel eating red-light foods after going on this diet, you weren't kidding!' – J

'On the couple days I made poor choices, I definitely noticed a difference in how I felt afterwards: depressed, lethargic and a bit nauseated. That combined with the minute weight loss has encouraged me that I need to avoid any deviations because they have such a trickle-down effect.' – Jenny

'Feeling well is a far better treat than whatever red-light food is on offer.' – Bernadette

The £5 cure is the food version of what immigrants (like me) used to call the '$1,000 cure'. Whenever a new arrival, after a long cold winter in Canada, started to pine for 'the old country', the cure was to get on a plane and go home for a week. All the reasons that originally persuaded the person to emigrate would come crashing back, and the thought of flying back to Canada began to look pretty good again.

With food, the cure costs less – say £5. But this is a motivator of last resort only – I certainly don't want to encourage people to abuse their bodies and feel awful! However, if you've been unceasingly pining for red-light foods, go out for lunch with some friends and order a high-Gi meal – perhaps a couple of slices of double-cheese pizza, a Coke and a brownie. Your mouth may enjoy it, but I guarantee that a couple hours later you'll be regretting the deviation!

Staying motivated is crucial to successful weight loss. It keeps you focused and on the green-light path, and it will get you through the pitfalls you'll encounter. Be sure to use all six of the above strategies – and you probably have a couple of your own that work well. Next week, we'll be discussing the relationship between weight and health – another highly motivating factor as you slim down to your ideal weight.

| Week 9 Weight | | Week 9 Waist | | Week 9 Hips | |

Week 9 Diary

_____

_____

_____

_____

_____

_____

_____

_____

_____

Optional week 9 meal plan

	Breakfast	Snack	Lunch
Mon	Homey Porridge (page 145) with chopped apple	Cranberry Cinnamon Bran Muffin (page 181)	Open-face chicken sandwich with lettuce, tomato and onion, and Basic Gi Salad (page 153)
Tue	Mini Breakfast Puffs (page 147)	Fruit yoghurt	Gi Pasta Salad (page 156)
Wed	Homemade Muesli (page 145) with skimmed milk and fruit yoghurt	Cranberry Cinnamon Bran Muffin (page 181)	1/2 wholemeal pitta with canned light tuna, lettuce, tomato and cucumber, and Basic Gi Salad (page 153)
Thu	Homey Porridge (page 145) with blueberries	Small apple and a glass of skimmed milk	Quick and Easy Chicken Noodle Soup (page 151) and Basic Gi Salad (page 153)
Fri	All-Bran with skimmed milk, peach slices and sliced almonds	Fruit yoghurt	Mixed Bean Salad (page 157)
Sat	Western Omelette (page 149)	1/2 food bar	Greek Salad (page 155)
Sun	Oatmeal Buttermilk Pancakes with Strawberries (page 146)	Orange and almonds	Tuscan White Bean Soup (page 151) and Basic Gi Salad (page 153)

Snack	Dinner	Snack
Laughing Cow Light cheese with high-fibre crispbread	Easy-Bake Lasagne (page 163) and Caesar Salad (page 154)	Mixed berries tossed in lime juice with soured cream
Hummus with carrot and celery sticks	Gi Fish Fillet (page 166), asparagus, carrots and new potatoes	Orange and almonds
Crunchy Chickpeas (page 181)	Chicken Curry (page 170) and Raita Salad (page 152)	Apple Pie Cookie (page 188) and a glass of skimmed milk
Fruit yoghurt	Vegetable Crumble (page 161) and Tabbouleh Salad (page 156)	1/2 food bar
Laughing Cow Light cheese with high-fibre crispbread	Chicken Fried Rice (page 170)	Mixed berries tossed in lime juice with soured cream
Hummus with carrot and celery sticks	Beef and Aubergine Chilli (page 176) and Basic Gi Salad (page 153)	Apple Pie Cookie (page 188) and a glass of skimmed milk
Fruit yoghurt	Pork Medallions Dijon (page 178), green beans, carrots and new potatoes	Piece of Plum Crumble (page 186)

Week 9 shopping list for meal plan

Produce

Almonds (whole and sliced)
Apples
Asparagus
Aubergines
Baby spinach
Bean sprouts
Blueberries or mixed summer berries
(fresh or frozen)
Broccoli
Carrots
Celery
Courgettes
Cranberries (dried)
Cucumbers
Fresh herbs (chives, mint, flat-leaf
parsley, sage, tarragon, thyme)
Garlic
Green beans
Kale
Leeks
Lemons
Lettuce (iceberg, leaf and Cos)
Mixed nuts
Mushrooms
Onions (yellow and red)
Oranges
Peaches (fresh or canned in juice or
water)
Peppers (red and green)
Potatoes (new, small)
Plums
Raisins
Sesame seeds
Spring onions
Strawberries
Sunflower seeds (shelled, unsalted)
Sweet potato
Tofu (firm)
Tomatoes (plum)

Deli

Feta cheese (light)
Hummus (light)
Kalamata olives
Parmesan cheese, grated

Bakery

High-fibre crispbread
100% stone-ground wholemeal
bread
Wholemeal pitta bread

Fish

Fish fillets (salmon or trout)

Meat

Back bacon
Beef mince (extra-lean)
Chicken breasts (boneless, skinless)
Pork tenderloins

Beans (legumes) and tinned vegetables

Chickpeas
Kidney beans (red and white)
Mixed beans
Tomatoes (chopped)
Tomatoes (plum)
Tomato puree

Pasta and sauces

Lasagne (wholemeal)
Fusilli or penne (wholemeal)
Small-shaped pasta (e.g. ditali or
tubetti)
Light tomato sauce (no added sugar)
Low-fat pasta sauce (no cheese or
meat in sauce)

Soup and tinned seafood and meat
Anchovy fillets
Chicken stock (low fat, low salt)
Tuna (light, in water)
Vegetable stock (low fat, low salt)

Grains and side dishes
Basmati rice
Brown rice
Bulgur wheat
Flaxseeds (ground)

International foods
Sesame oil
Soy sauce (low salt)
Tahini

Cooking oil, vinegar, salad dressings and pickles
Cooking oil spray (vegetable or olive oil)
Dijon mustard
Mayonnaise (fat-free)
Oil (vegetable and extra-virgin olive)
Red wine vinegar
Worcestershire sauce

Snacks
Apple sauce (unsweetened)
Food bars (e.g. Slim-Fast)

Baking
Baking powder
Bicarbonate of soda
Cornflour
Oat bran

Spices (ground cardamom, cayenne pepper, chilli powder, ground cinnamon, ground cumin, curry powder, ground ginger, ground nutmeg, dried oregano, black pepper, red pepper flakes, salt, dried thyme)
Splenda
Vanilla extract
Wheat bran
Wheat germ
Wholemeal flour

Breakfast foods
All-Bran cereal
Oatmeal (large-flake oats)

Beverages
White wine

Dairy
Buttermilk
Cheddar cheese (low fat)
Cottage cheese (low fat)
Fruit yoghurt (non-fat with sweetener)
Laughing Cow cheese (light)
Margarine (soft, non-hydrogenated, light)
Milk (skimmed)
Mozzarella cheese (low fat)
Plain yoghurt (non-fat)
Soured cream (light)
Whole Omega-3 eggs

Frozen foods
Mixed berries
Peas (or fresh)

Week 10 Your Health – What's at Stake

This week's topic follows from last week's discussion of motivation, since one of the top motivating factors for losing weight, as we saw in Week 1, is wanting to achieve better health. The connection between being overweight and being at increased risk for certain diseases is well established. Let's look at these risks in turn.

Heart disease and stroke

Given that I was the president of the Heart and Stroke Foundation of Ontario for fifteen years, it is hardly surprising that I'm starting with these diseases. However, there is a more important reason: heart disease and stroke cause 40 per cent of North American deaths. Remarkably this is evidence of progress. When I first joined the Foundation, the figure was close to 50 per cent. This is a good news/bad news story. The good news is that advances in surgery, drug therapies and emergency services have saved many lives. The bad news is that twice as many deaths could have been averted if only we had reduced our weight, exercised regularly and quit smoking. Though the smoking rate for adults has dropped sharply (unfortunately, we cannot say the same for teens), we are eating more and exercising less, leading inevitably to a more obese and unhealthy population. It's been calculated that if we led even a moderate lifestyle, we could halve the carnage from these diseases. Though heart disease, like most cancers, is primarily a disease of old age, nearly half of those who suffer heart attacks are under the age of sixty-five.

A familiar refrain that I have heard many times is: 'Why worry? If I have a heart attack, today's medicine will save me.' It might well save you from immediate death, but the heart is permanently damaged after an attack. The heart cannot repair itself because its cells do not reproduce. After the damage sustained during a heart attack, the heart has to work harder to compensate – but it never can. It slowly degenerates under this stress, and patients finally 'drown' as blood circulation fails and the lungs fill with liquid. Congestive heart failure is a dreadful way to die, so make sure you do everything you can to avoid having a heart attack in the first place.

The simple fact is that the more overweight you are, the more likely you will suffer a heart attack or stroke. The two key factors that link heart disease and stroke to diet are cholesterol and hypertension (high blood pressure). High blood pressure puts more stress on the arterial system, causing it to age and deteriorate more rapidly, and ultimately leads to arterial damage, blood clots and heart attack or stroke. Excess weight has a major bearing on high blood pressure. One Canadian study found that obese adults, aged eighteen to fifty-five, had a five to thirteen times greater risk of hypertension. A further study demonstrated that a lower fat diet coupled with a major increase in fruits and vegetables (eight to ten servings a day) lowered blood pressure. The moral: lose weight and eat more fruits and vegetables to help reduce your blood pressure levels. In other words, eat the green-light way.

Cholesterol is essential to your body's metabolism. However, high cholesterol is a problem as it's the key ingredient in the plaque that can build up in your arteries, eventually cutting off the blood supply to your heart (causing heart attack) or your brain (leading to stroke). To make things more complicated, there are two forms of cholesterol: HDL (good) cholesterol and LDL (bad) cholesterol. The idea is to boost the HDL level while depressing the LDL level. (Remember it this way: HDL is Heart's Delight Level and LDL is Leads to Death Level.) The villain in raising LDL levels is saturated fat, which is usually solid at room temperature and is found primarily in meat and whole milk products. Conversely, polyunsaturated and monounsaturated fats not only lower LDL levels but also boost HDL. The moral: make sure some fat is included in your diet, but make sure it's the right fat (see page 9).

Diabetes

Diabetes is the kissing cousin of heart disease in that more people die from heart complications arising from diabetes than from diabetes alone. And diabetes rates are skyrocketing: they are expected to double in the next ten years. The principal causes of the most common form of diabetes, Type 2, are obesity and lack of exercise, and the current epidemic is strongly correlated to the obesity trend. The most dramatic illustration of this link appears in Canada's Native population, where in some communities diabetes affects nearly half the adults. Before the Europeans colonised North America, the Native peoples lived in a state of feast or famine. When there was an abundance of food, plant or animal, it was stored in the body as fat. In lean times, such as winter, the body depleted these fat supplies. As a result, their bodies developed a 'thrift gene', with those who stored and utilised their food most effectively being the survivors – a classic Darwinian example of survival of the fittest. When you take away famine and the need to hunt or to harvest food – that is, the need to exercise – and replace it with a trip to the super-market whenever food is required, the result is inevitable: a massive increase in obesity and, with it, diabetes.

Foods with a low Gi rating, which release sugar more slowly into the blood-stream, appear to play a major role in helping diabetics control their disease. Thus the Gi Diet provides an opportunity both to lose weight and to assist in the management of the disease. In its magazine, Dialogue, the Canadian

Diabetes Association selected the Gi Diet as its diet of choice. Because protein and fat affect a food's Gi rating, diabetics should be particularly careful about eating the right balance of green-light protein, carbohydrates and fat at every meal and snack. Prevention, however, is far preferable, so keep going with your green-light programme and continue to slim down.

Cancer

There is increasing research evidence that diets high in saturated fat are linked to certain cancers, particularly prostate and colorectal cancer. A recent global report by the American Institute for Cancer Research concluded that 30 to 40 per cent of cancers are directly linked to dietary choices. Its key recommendation is that we choose a diet that includes a variety of vegetables, fruit and grains, and is low in saturated fat – in a nutshell, the Gi Diet.

Alzheimer's Disease

As with cancer, there is increasing evidence linking certain dementias, particularly Alzheimer's, with fat intake. A recent US study showed a 40 per cent increase in Alzheimer's disease for those who ate a diet high in saturated fat.

Abdominal fat and health

Although your BMI is a measure of body fat based on your height and weight, it is not necessarily the best guide to assessing your health risk. Where you're storing the fat is the real issue. The results of a recent worldwide survey involving 27,000 people showed that people who carried their extra weight around their waists (apple shaped) were at far greater risk of disease than those who carried their weight lower down on their hips (pear shaped). From the study came this table showing the risk of disease based on weight and waist measurement.

A 'beer belly' is not just extra weight. Rather it is an active, living part of your body. Once it has formed sufficient mass, it behaves like an organ such as the liver, heart or kidney, except that it pumps out a dangerous combination of free fatty acids and proteins. The fact is that abdominal fat has many of the characteristics of a huge tumour. A waist measurement of 35 inches or more for women and 40 inches or more for men puts you in the High Risk category for developing heart disease, stroke, hypertension (high blood pressure) and certain types of cancer – breast, uterus, colon for women, and prostate and colon for men.

A further refinement, and an even better predictor of your health, is your waist-to-hip ratio. This is calculated by dividing your waist measurement by your hip measurement. A healthy ratio for women is 0.85 or below, and 0.95 or below for men. If you are a woman with a hip measurement of 42 inches and a waist measurement of 38 inches, your waist to hip ratio is 0.90, which puts you at risk. If your hip measurement was still 42 inches but your waist was only 34 inches, your ratio would be an acceptable 0.80.

WEIGHT	BMI	WAIST	WAIST
		Women less than 35" Men less than 40"	Women 35" plus MEN 40"plus
Normal	18.0–24.9	No risk increase	No risk increase
Overweight	25.0–29.9	Increased risk	High risk
Obese	30.0–39.9	High risk	Very high risk

Joint degeneration

Finally, there is the issue of joint degeneration caused by excessive weight loading. Just recently the Canadian Institute of Health published a survey of knee and hip replacements performed in Canada between 2004 and 2005. It showed that not only had the number of operations nearly doubled over the past ten years, but also overweight patients accounted for a startling 87 per cent of knee replacements and 74 per cent of hip replacements.

If you want to reduce your risk for these diseases and keep your joints intact, then keep up your green-light diet. I can't think of a better motivator.

Week 10 Weight　　**Week 10 Waist**　　**Week 10 Hips**

Week 10 Diary

Optional week 10 meal plan

	Breakfast	Snack	Lunch
Mon	Homey Porridge (page 145) with chopped apple	Carrot Muffin (page 182)	Open-face lean deli ham sandwich with lettuce, tomato, red pepper and wholegrain mustard, and Basic Gi Salad (page 153)
Tue	Mini Breakfast Puffs (page 147)	Fruit yoghurt	Waldorf Chicken and Rice Salad (page 157)
Wed	Homemade Muesli (page 145) with skimmed milk and fruit yoghurt	Carrot Muffin (page 182)	Cottage cheese with apple and grapes, and Basic Gi Salad (page 153)
Thu	Homey Porridge (page 145) with berries	Small apple and a glass of skimmed milk	Minestrone Soup (page 150) and Basic Gi Salad (page 153)
Fri	All-Bran with skimmed milk, peach slices and sliced almonds	Fruit yoghurt	1/2 wholemeal pitta with deli turkey, lettuce, tomato and cucumber, and Basic Gi Salad (page 153)
Sat	Italian Omelette (page 148) or Homey Porridge (page 145)	1/2 food bar	Crab Salad in Tomato Shells (page 158)
Sun	Cinnamon French Toast (page 146) with back bacon	Orange and almonds	Ham and Lentil Soup (page 152) and Basic Gi Salad (page 153)

Week 10 shopping list for meal plan

Produce
Almonds (whole and sliced)
Apples
Asparagus
Baby spinach
Blueberries or mixed summer berries (fresh or frozen)
Broccoli
Carrots
Celery
Courgettes (yellow)
Cucumbers
Fresh herbs (basil, chives, coriander, flat-leaf parsley)
Garlic
Ginger root
Grapes

Green beans
Lemon
Lettuce (leaf and Cos)
Limes
Mangetout
Mushrooms
Onions (yellow and red)
Oranges
Peaches (fresh or canned in juice or water)
Pecans
Peppers (red and green)
Potatoes (new, small)
Raisins
Raspberries
Sesame seeds
Spring onions

Snack	Dinner	Snack
Laughing Cow Light cheese with high-fibre crispbread	Fettuccine Primavera (page 159) and Caesar Salad (page 154)	Mixed berries tossed in lime juice with soured cream
Hummus with carrot and celery sticks	Ginger-Wasabi Halibut (page 167), Cold Noodle Salad with Cucumber and Sesame (page 155), snow peas and carrots	Orange and almonds
Cottage cheese (light) with peach slices	Chicken Tarragon with Mushrooms (page 173), broccoli and basmati rice	Pecan Brownie (page 189) and a glass of skimmed milk
Crunchy Chickpeas (page 181)	Meatloaf (page 175), green beans, carrots and new potatoes	½ food bar
Laughing Cow Light cheese with high-fibre crispbread	Bean and Onion Pizza (page 162)	Mixed berries tossed in lime juice with soured cream
Hummus with carrot and celery sticks	Grilled Tuna with Chimichurri Sauce (page 168), asparagus and new potatoes	Pecan Brownie (page 189) and a glass of skimmed milk
Fruit yoghurt	Orange Chicken with Almonds (page 172), green beans and basmati rice	Slice of Apple Raspberry Coffee Cake (page 187)

Strawberries
Sunflower seeds, shelled and unsalted
Tofu (firm)
Tomatoes (large beefsteak and plum)
Tomatoes (sun-dried)
Walnuts

Deli
Feta cheese (light)
Hummus (light)
Lean deli ham
Lean deli turkey
Parmesan cheese, grated

Bakery
High-fibre crispbread
100% stone-ground wholemeal bread
Wholemeal pitta bread

Fish
Frozen crab
Halibut fillets
Tuna steaks (½-inch thick)

Meat
Back bacon
Beef mince (extra-lean)
Chicken breasts (boneless, skinless)

Beans (legumes) and tinned vegetables
Chickpeas
Kidney beans (red and white)
Lentils
Tomatoes (plum)
Tomato purée

Pasta and sauces
Capellini or spaghetti (wholemeal)
Fettuccini or linguine (wholemeal)
Low fat pasta sauce (no cheese or meat in sauce)
Small-shaped pasta (ditali or tubetti)

Soup and tinned seafood and meat
Anchovy fillets
Chicken stock (low fat, low salt)
Vegetable stock (low fat, low salt)

Grains and side dishes
Basmati rice
Flaxseeds (ground)

International foods
Mirin (or sweet sherry)
Rice vinegar
Soy sauce (low sodium)
Sesame seeds (toasted)
Tahini
Wasabi powder

Cooking oil, vinegar, salad dressings and pickles
Buttermilk salad dressing (low fat, low sugar)
Cooking oil spray (vegetable or olive oil)
Dijon mustard
Oil (vegetable and extra-virgin olive)
Red wine vinegar
Wholegrain mustard
Worcestershire sauce

Snacks
Food bars (e.g. Slim-Fast)

Baking
Active dry yeast
Baking powder
Bicarbonate of soda
Brown-sugar substitute
Cornflour
Oat bran
Spices (black pepper, cayenne pepper, cinnamon, ground ginger, ground nutmeg, dried oregano, red-pepper flakes, salt, dried tarragon, dried thyme)
Splenda
Unsweetened cocoa powder
Vanilla extract
Wheat bran
Wheat germ
Wholemeal flour

Breakfast foods
All-Bran cereal
Oatmeal (large-flake oats)

Beverages
Tomato juice
Vegetable cocktail juice
Vermouth or white wine

Dairy
Buttermilk
Cottage cheese (low fat)
Fruit yoghurt (non-fat with sweetener)
Laughing Cow cheese (light)
Margarine (soft, non-hydrogenated, light)
Milk (skimmed)
Mozzarella cheese (low fat)
Soured cream (low fat)
Whole omega-3 eggs

Frozen foods
Mixed berries
Peas (or fresh)

Week 11 Holidays and Special Events

Holidays are undoubtedly the most difficult times of the year for anyone trying to lose weight. While it may not actually be the holiday season when you come to this chapter, its advice can be applied to any sort of celebratory occasion, such as an anniversary or wedding. And of course, you can always turn to this chapter when you are faced with the challenge of an approaching holiday. Celebrations like Christmas and Easter all have an abundance of food, and much of it is red-light. Many people gain weight as they indulge in the feasts at family get-togethers, office cocktail parties and neighbours' open houses, but it doesn't have to be this way. You can enjoy all the festivities and still stay mostly in the green. While it is probably unrealistic to expect you will lose weight during holiday time, your goal should be to not put on any more weight – after all, you've worked hard to achieve the progress you've made and you don't want to undo it! Here are my suggestions for navigating this dangerous terrain.

The Cocktail Party

Never go to a cocktail party hungry or you are likely to overindulge. Instead, have a small green-light meal or snack before heading out. A bowl of high-fibre green-light cereal will do the trick.

Once you arrive, be sure to get yourself a drink. It's important to always have a drink in hand at a cocktail party; if you don't, someone will probably pass you one that you haven't chosen – or you'll be looking for nibbles to occupy your empty hands. Soda water with a twist of lime or diet caffeine-free soft drinks are green-light choices. If you really would like an alcoholic beverage, bypass the beer and fancy cocktails, which are caloric nightmares, and instead choose a white wine spritzer or a glass of red wine. Try to limit yourself to one, and then switch to soda water.

Be sure to consume any alcohol with food to slow the rate at which you metabolise it. Look for green-light snacks such as mixed raw vegetables with low-fat dips such as hummus and salsa, lean sliced turkey and deli ham, shrimp (not breaded), smoked salmon, and fruit. Do not station yourself beside the bowls of nuts and olives – they may be green-light but restricting yourself to a small handful will prove difficult.

The holiday dinner

It's easy to make your traditional festive meal green-light with some minor adjustments. Here are some guidelines:

Soup: Start the meal with a delicious, homemade green-light soup made with stock, vegetables and fresh herbs.

Salad: Always serve a large salad with homemade green-light dressing. Make it more festive by adding toasted pecans and a sprinkling of dried cranberries or crumbled blue cheese. Ruth makes a delicious salad of Cos lettuce, sliced strawberries and raspberry vinaigrette. Super easy and very pretty. The salad can be served before the main course to help fill you up, or as one of the side dishes.

Turkey: Prepare a roast turkey and eat the white breast meat – without the skin, of course. Instead of making stuffing with bread crumbs, use wild or basmati rice flavoured with apples or mushrooms, celery, onions and herbs.

Vegetables: There is a wide array of green-light vegetable dishes to choose from. Try roasted, braised or steamed vegetables in various combinations with flavourings of lemon, balsamic vinegar or herbs.

Sweet potatoes: If you consider sweet potatoes an essential part of your holiday feast, then go ahead and have them, but instead of adding brown sugar or maple syrup, try ground ginger, light non-hydrogenated margarine, pepper and hot water if needed.

Cranberry sauce: If you make cranberry sauce, replace sugar with Splenda. Ruth always adds some chopped orange and slivered almonds for extra flavour and crunch.

Dessert: Dessert can always be part of a green-light meal. All of my books contain recipes for delicious desserts. A sweet treat to end your holiday dinner could be a low-fat, no-sugar-added ice cream, fresh berries with sweetened yoghurt cheese, poached pears or a fruit crumble.

Hosting the holiday dinner yourself will obviously give you far greater control over the food. However, as a visitor you can still exert some influence by bringing a green-light side dish or dessert and serving yourself. Compose your plate as you would at home: vegetables on half the plate, rice or pasta on one-quarter and a source of protein on the other one-quarter. Pass on the rolls and mashed potatoes – have extra vegetables instead. If you wish, you can allow yourself a concession by having a small serving of dessert. If you don't have much of a sweet tooth, you might prefer to have a glass of wine instead. Try not to indulge in both.

Here are some ways e-Clinic participants dealt with the holidays:

'The newest strategy for our Christmas preparation is to focus on establishing new traditions with decorating and doing specific things together instead of the classics from my past that revolved around Christmas treats, such as Toblerone, Chocolate Oranges, Christmas cake, and so on.' – Bernadette

'Thanksgiving went fairly well, with boiled new potatoes instead of mashed and smaller portions of white meat only and no seconds.' – Ross

'I was pleasantly surprised to get on the scales this morning and find I still weighed the same! One of the things I noticed yesterday was I was not left with that sick, stuffed feeling after the Thanksgiving meal! My biggest challenge was not tasting as I cooked the meal and deciding what to do with the leftovers, which I didn't want to waste. Would I rather they go to my waist? Not! I gave away over half of them. We will have a few sensible meals out of the healthier ones. Some I simply dumped! Yay!' – Diane

'Events such as Thanksgiving, Halloween and birthdays were always a "free" ticket to overeat for me – it was almost as though it was expected. This time was different. I still enjoyed the food and celebrations, but when tempted to slide I thought, "Is it worth having to wait another week or two or more to get to my goal?" I think more now about what I am going to eat and why, especially if I'm out. I realise now what a lot of junk we feed ourselves. I wish that parents of young children would recognise this and take action, because they don't truly understand (and can't unless they have been there and lived it themselves) the impact that being overweight will have on their child emotionally, psychologically and physically, and the social stigma they will face.' – Kathy

'This weekend was the weekend for us for holiday parties. Friday night, Saturday lunch, Saturday night and Sunday lunch, followed by concert and dessert reception ... I made myself a deal to cope with the events (I had no control over the food available): If I could eat mostly green- and some yellow-light foods, I could have a drink or two. If there were only yellow- or red-light foods available, it was club soda and lime for me.' – Karen

Week 11 Weight	☐	Week 11 Waist	☐	Week 11 Hips	☐

Week 11 Diary

_____

_____

_____

_____

_____

_____

_____

_____

_____

_____

Optional week 11 meal plan

	Breakfast	Snack	Lunch
Mon	Homey Porridge (page 145) with chopped apple	Apple Bran Muffin (page 182)	Open-face chicken sandwich with lettuce, tomato and onion, and Basic Gi Salad (page 153)
Tue	Mini Breakfast Puffs (page 147)	Fruit yoghurt	Gi Pasta Salad (page 156)
Wed	Homemade Muesli (page 145) with skimmed milk and fruit yoghurt	Apple Bran Muffin (page 182)	1/2 wholemeal pitta with canned light tuna, lettuce, tomato and cucumber, and Basic Gi Salad (page 153)
Thu	Homey Porridge (page 145) with blueberries	Small apple and a glass of skimmed milk	Quick and Easy Chicken Noodle Soup (page 151) and Basic Gi Salad (page 153)
Fri	All-Bran with skimmed milk, peach slices and sliced almonds	Fruit yoghurt	Mixed Bean Salad (page 157)
Sat	Vegetarian Omelette (page 149) or Homey Porridge (page 145)	1/2 food bar	Greek Salad (page 155)
Sun	Oatmeal Buttermilk Pancakes with Strawberries (page 146)	Orange and almonds	Tuscan White Bean Soup (page 151) and Basic Gi Salad (page 153)

Snack	Dinner	Snack
Laughing Cow Light cheese with high-fibre crispbread	Rigatoni with Mini-Meat Balls (page 177) and Caesar Salad (page 154)	Mixed berries tossed in lime juice with soured cream
Hummus with carrot and celery sticks	Citrus-Poached Haddock (page 167), green beans and new potatoes	Orange and almonds
Fruit yoghurt	Chicken Jambalaya (page 172) and broccoli	Creamy Lemon Square (page 190) and a glass of skimmed milk
Crunchy Chickpeas (page 181)	Barley Risotto with Leeks, Lemon and Peas (page 160) and Tabbouleh Salad (page 156)	½ food bar
Laughing Cow Light cheese with high-fibre crispbread	Thai Red Curry Prawn Pasta (page 166)	Mixed berries tossed in lime juice with soured cream
Hummus with carrot and celery sticks	Zesty Barbecued Chicken (page 174), Tangy Red and Green Coleslaw (page 153) and new potatoes	Creamy Lemon Square (page 190) and a glass of skimmed milk
Yoghurt with peach slices	Pork Tenderloin with Apple Compote (page 180), Brussels sprouts, carrots and new potatoes	Piece of Berry Crumble (page 185)

Week 11 shopping list for meal plan

Produce

Almonds (whole and sliced)
Apples
Aubergines
Blueberries or mixed summer berries (fresh or frozen)
Broccoli
Brussels sprouts
Cabbage (green and red)
Carrots
Celery
Courgettes
Cucumbers
Currants
Fresh herbs (chives, coriander, flat-leaf parsley, mint, rosemary, sage and thyme)
Garlic
Green beans
Kale
Leek
Lemons
Lettuce (leaf, iceberg and Cos)
Limes
Mushrooms
Onions (yellow and red)
Oranges
Peaches (fresh or canned in juice or water)
Pecans
Peppers (red and green)
Potatoes (new, small)
Spring onions
Strawberries
Sunflower seeds, shelled and unsalted
Tomatoes (plum)

Deli

Feta cheese (light)
Hummus (light)
Kalamata olives
Parmesan cheese, grated

Bakery

High-fibre crispbread
100% stone-ground wholemeal bread
Wholemeal pitta bread

Fish

Haddock fillets
Shrimp (large raw)

Meat

Chicken breasts (boneless, skinless)
Lean chicken or turkey mince
Pork tenderloin

Beans (legumes) and tinned vegetables

Chickpeas
Kidney beans (red and white)
Mixed beans
Tomatoes (plum)
Tomatoes (stewed)
Tomato puree

Pasta and sauces

Fusilli or penne (wholemeal)
Macaroni or small shells (wholemeal)
Rigatoni (wholemeal)
Small-shaped pasta (e.g., ditali or tubetti)
Spaghetti or linguine (wholemeal)
Light tomato sauce

Soup and tinned seafood and meat

Anchovy fillets
Chicken stock (low fat, low sodium)
Tuna (light, in water)
Vegetable stock (low fat, low sodium)

Grains and side dishes
Barley
Brown rice
Bulgur
Flaxseeds (ground)

International foods
Tahini
Thai red curry paste

Cooking oil, vinegar, salad dressings and pickles
Cider vinegar
Cooking oil spray (vegetable or olive oil)
Dijon mustard
Mayonnaise (fat free)
Oil (vegetable and extra-virgin olive)
Red wine vinegar
Worcestershire sauce

Snacks
Apple sauce (unsweetened)
Food bars (e.g. Slim-Fast)

Baking
Baking powder
Bicarbonate of soda
Brown-sugar substitute
Cornflour
Ground almonds
Oat bran
Spices (ground allspice, bay leaves, black pepper, cayenne pepper, celery seeds, chilli powder, ground cinnamon, ground cloves, ground cumin, dried oregano, dried sage, salt and dried thyme)

Splenda
Vanilla extract
Wheat bran
Wheat germ
Wholemeal flour

Breakfast foods
All-Bran cereal
Oatmeal (large-flake oats)

Beverages
Apple juice (unsweetened)
Dry white wine (or vermouth)

Dairy
Buttermilk
Cheddar cheese (low fat)
Fruit yoghurt (non-fat with sweetener)
Laughing Cow cheese (light)
Margarine (soft, non-hydrogenated, light)
Milk (skimmed)
Orange juice (unsweetened)
Soured cream (low fat)
Whole omega-3 eggs

Frozen foods
Frozen apple juice concentrate
Mixed berries
Peas (or fresh)

Week 12 Exercise

As the e-Clinic progressed and participants lost a considerable amount of weight and found their energy levels increasing, many decided to get involved in regular exercise.

'Now that eating is becoming more routine, I want to establish an exercise programme. I think this will be important.' – Lynn

'I can almost see the 100s and I am dying to get there! ... I joined Curves (a fitness club) yesterday.' – Beverley

'I am down below what I have been for the past seven years. That is encouraging and I know I will continue the good eating habits I have practised for the last three months. I also know I am at a place where I need to increase my daily exercise.' – Diane

'When my baby was six months old I tried jogging but was discouraged when I felt a lot of pain in my shins. This past Thursday I tried it again and had great success. I have jogged almost every day so far.' – Tammy

There are many benefits to exercising. Regular exercise will contribute significantly to your health by reducing your risk of heart disease, stroke, diabetes and osteoporosis; maintaining your muscle mass and tone as you age; and, over the long term, accelerating or maintaining your weight loss. In the United States, the National Weight Loss Registry is tracking some 3000 people who have lost over two stone or more and kept it off for six years. One thing they have in common is that they are very active and exercise every day. Although exercise is of limited value in helping achieve your weight-loss target, it becomes a critical factor in helping maintain your weight and health for the rest of your life. And believe it or not, exercise can become addictive. I tend to become irritable and edgy if I'm not getting my daily exercise fix – or so Ruth tells me. Initially, it can be hard to get out there and hit the sidewalk or gym, but stick with it – the fun will kick in eventually.

Before we go any further, we should define exactly what we mean by exercise. There are three basic types of exercise, each working with the others.

Types of Exercise

Aerobic

Aerobic exercise gets your heart and lungs working harder. Aerobic exercise, such as walking, jogging, biking, swimming, hiking and so on, will have the most impact on your overall weight and health.

Strength

Strength training is particularly important as we move into middle age and beyond because of the steady reduction in muscle mass that accompanies aging. Starting at the age of twenty-five, the body loses 2 per cent of its muscle mass each decade, a process that accelerates to 6 to 8 per cent as we move into our senior years.

Exercising muscles on a regular basis minimises or reverses the loss. And why is that important? Because the larger your muscles, the more energy (calories) they use. When you're at rest, or even asleep in bed, your muscles are using energy. So keeping or building muscle mass really helps you burn calories and lose weight.

Though regular exercise will help minimise muscle loss, it is through resistance exercises that we actually build muscle mass. Resistance exercises involve fixed or free weights, elastic bands or even your own body weight; pushing your hands together as hard as you can is a form of resistance exercise. You don't have to join a gym or work out with massive barbells. A few simple exercises, easily done at home, will do wonders to restore or tone those flabby muscles.

Stretching

Again this is a significant issue as we age and lose flexibility in our joints, tendons and ligaments. Loss of flexibility reduces our ability to do either aerobic or strength training, both of which depend on healthy joints and tissues. In older people, this loss of flexibility can lead to falls and hip fractures. So although stretching may seem like a 'frill', it is central to the whole fitness picture. Stretching exercises will also give you the biggest bang for your buck in terms of immediate payout. Within just a week, you can increase your flexibility by over 100 per cent. Both aerobic and strength training can actually make you less flexible if you don't stretch those muscle ligaments and tendons. That's why you always see athletes warming up and down with stretching exercises. Always include stretching in your exercise programme.

Now let's review your options.

Outdoor activities

Walking

This is by far the simplest and, for most people, the easiest exercise programme to start and maintain. For adults, thirty minutes a day, seven days a week, should be the target. If you do an hour-long walk one day of the weekend, you can take a day off during the week. We're talking about brisk walking, neither speed walking nor ambling along. Imagine you're late for an appointment, and keep that pace. You should increase your heart and breathing rates, but never to the point where you lack the breath to talk with a partner.

You don't need any special clothing or equipment, except a pair of comfortable cushioned shoes or running shoes. Walking is rarely boring since you can change routes and watch the world go by. Walk with your spouse, child or friend for company and mutual support, or go solo and commune with nature and your own thoughts. I prefer to walk on my own in the morning, which is when I do my best thinking. This is not surprising when you realise how much extra oxygen-fresh blood is pumping through the brain.

A great idea for working people is to incorporate walking into the daily commute. I used to get off the bus three stops early on my way to and from work. Those three stops are equal to about one and a half miles, so I was walking about three miles per day! If you drive to work, try parking your car a few blocks away and walk to your job. You may even find cheaper parking. Gradually increase the distance and your exercise. Who knows, you may eventually be able to walk to work. Think of the savings in petrol and parking fees!

Jogging

This is similar to walking, but you need the proper footwear to protect joints from damage. Jogging approximately doubles the number of calories burned in the same period of time as walking: 400 calories for jogging versus 200 for brisk walking over a 30-minute period. While walking, try jogging for a few yards and see if it is for you. Jogging increases your heart rate, which is great for heart health. Like all muscles, the heart thrives on exercise so, in general, the more the better. If jogging suits you, then this could be the simplest and most effective method of exercise as it can be done anywhere, and is inexpensive.

Hiking

Another variation on walking is cross-country hiking. Because this usually involves different kinds of terrain, especially hills and valleys, you use more calories, about 50 per cent more than for brisk walking. Try hauling 10 to 15 stone up a hill and you'll get some idea of the extra effort your body has to make.

Cycling

Like walking, jogging and hiking, cycling is a fun way to burn calories, and it is almost as effective as jogging (for people with low-back or knee problems, it can be preferable). Other than the cost of the bike and helmet, it's inexpensive and can be done almost anywhere, with lights and reflectors for night riding, of course.

Sports

Although most sports are terrific calorie burners, they usually cannot be part of a regular routine. Most of them require other people, equipment and facilities. But they can provide a boost to your regular fitness and exercise programme. Such popular sports as tennis, basketball, soccer, softball and golf (no golf cart, please) are excellent additions to a basic exercise programme. However, they're no substitute for a five- to seven-day-a-week regular schedule.

Indoor activities

Many of you will be muttering by now about how this would be fine advice if we lived in California. But many of us must contend with either frigid, snowy winters or hot, humid summers, which limit outdoor activities.

The alternatives are either to organise a home gym or join a fitness club. The advantage of clubs is that they offer a wide range of sophisticated equipment, with instruction and advice from staff. Clubs are also social, and some people find they need group motivation to work out with enthusiasm. YMCAs/YWCAs and some community centres also offer special programmes for elderly people, new mothers, and those with special needs; some provide subsidies for people who can't afford the membership fees. Many centres offer free fitness classes too.

If a fitness club isn't convenient or those Lycra-clad young things make you uncomfortable, you can always set up an exercise area at home. The best and least expensive piece of equipment is a stationary bike. The latest models work on magnetic resistance rather than the old friction strap around the flywheel. This gives a smoother action, with better tension adjustment. Most important, they are quiet, which is crucial if you want to be able to listen to music or watch TV. You can easily pay in the thousands for a bike with all the fancy trimmings, but the £250 to £300 machines will work fine. Just be sure you choose one that has smooth, adjustable tension; then, pop in that late-night movie or your favourite soap and get pedalling. You'll be amazed how quickly the minutes fly by. Twenty minutes on the bike consumes the same number of calories as thirty minutes of brisk walking.

If biking is not for you, try a treadmill. These can be expensive, and beware of the lower-end models that cannot take the pounding. Expect to pay about £1,000 and up. Make sure the incline of the track can be raised and lowered for a better workout. Both treadmills and bikes can simulate outdoor walking, jogging, hiking or biking in the comfort of your own home. I use both of these machines but have added a cross-country ski machine, which has the advantage of working the upper body as well. Ski machines are generally less expensive than treadmills, but cost more than stationary bikes. They also burn a lot of calories (similar to the amount burned when jogging) because they use the arms and shoulders as well as the legs. Ski machines are almost the perfect all-body workout machine. There are several other specialised options, such as stair climber machines, elliptical walkers and rowing machines, but they're not for everyone. Many are also quite expensive, so try them out first at a fitness club or with a cooperative retailer.

Strength training

It's now time to pay attention to rebuilding your muscle mass. Remember that after age forty, you may lose between four and six pounds of muscle every decade, which is usually replaced with flab. That's four to six pounds of calorie-consuming muscle. Muscles burn energy even when idle, and bigger muscles consume more energy than smaller muscles. So muscles come in handy for losing or maintaining weight.

Resistance-training equipment can range from the complex and expensive to a £5 rubber band. Home gyms, with prices that begin at about a hundred pounds, are a popular option. For most people, however, there are cheaper, simpler methods, such as a set of free weights or (my own preference) rubber exercise bands. Dyna-Band and Thera-Band are two popular choices. I like using Thera-Bands, which come in varying thicknesses that offer increasing levels of resistance as you regain and build your muscle strength.

Weights and these resistance rubber bands are available at many fitness exercise equipment retailers and surgical supply stores. Try a few resistance exercises, concentrating on the larger muscle groups – your legs, arms and upper chest. These are the muscles that will give you the biggest bang by burning up the most calories. Resistance exercises should complement your regular exercise regimen, not replace it. Committing to both types of exercise will produce far better results than either one alone. Resistance exercises are best done every other day, leaving time for your muscles to recuperate.

Pilates

I've recently become a Pilates enthusiast. Originally, it was recommended by my physiotherapist to strengthen my back and prevent my disc problem from recurring. However, this very precise system of exercises does a lot more than just that. It's a series of floor exercises – no equipment needed – that both strengthen and stretch your muscles, especially the core muscles in your back and around your waist, which are essential for good posture. It's great for any level of fitness and at any age.

Yoga and tai chi

Yoga comes in different styles: hatha, kundalini, kripalu, ashtanga, bikram and others. If you're new to yoga, the best choice is hatha, which teaches you simple postures that will keep you supple, offer relaxation techniques and improve your breathing and circulation. Ashtanga is trendy nowadays, but it is more aerobic and demanding. Kundalini focuses more on energising breathing techniques and meditation. But in any form, this ancient practice has much to offer, especially to anyone taking up exercise in middle age.

Tai chi is another Eastern discipline that is gentle, promoting flexibility, balance and energy. It features a series of flowing postures, done standing, that many people like to practise early in the morning, outdoors. Tai chi keeps the joints and tendons supple, and offers a peaceful, revitalising form of activity that can carry you into old age. Instructional DVDs or videos are available for those who want to learn or practise yoga or Tai Chi at home.

Whether you take up walking, hockey, dance lessons or nature hikes, make sure it is an activity you enjoy. If you take pleasure from your exercise you are more likely to do it.

Week 12 Weight	Week 12 Waist	Week 12 Hips

Week 12 Diary

Optional week 12 meal plan

	Breakfast	Snack	Lunch
Mon	Homey Porridge (page 145) with chopped apple	Wholemeal Fruit Scone (page 183)	Open-face lean deli ham sandwich with lettuce, tomato, red pepper and wholegrain mustard, and Basic Gi Salad (page 153)
Tue	Mini Breakfast Puffs (page 147)	Fruit yoghurt	Waldorf Chicken and Rice Salad (page 157)
Wed	Homemade Muesli (page 145) with skimmed milk and fruit yoghurt	Wholemeal Fruit Scone (page 183)	Cottage cheese with apple and grapes, and Basic Gi Salad (page 153)
Thu	Homey Porridge (page 145) with blueberries	Small apple and a glass of skimmed milk	Minestrone Soup (page 150) and Basic Gi Salad (page 153)
Fri	All-Bran with skimmed milk, peach slices and sliced almonds	Fruit yoghurt	½ wholemeal pitta with deli turkey, lettuce, tomato and cucumber, and Basic Gi Salad (page 153)
Sat	Back Bacon Omelette (page 149) or Homey Porridge (page 145)	½ food bar	Crab Salad in Tomato Shells (page 158)
Sun	Cinnamon French Toast (page 146) with back bacon	Orange and almonds	Ham and Lentil Soup (page 152) and Basic Gi Salad (page 153)

Week 12 shopping list for meal plan

Produce
Alfalfa sprouts (optional)
Almonds (whole and sliced)
Apples
Asparagus
Aubergines
Baby spinach
Blueberries or mixed summer berries (fresh or frozen)
Broccoli
Carrots
Celery
Cucumbers
Dried apricots
Fresh herbs (basil, chives, coriander, flat-leaf parsley, mint, tarragon)
Garlic
Grapes
Green beans
Lemons
Lettuce (leaf)
Limes
Mushrooms
Onions (yellow and red)
Oranges
Peaches (fresh or canned in juice or water)
Pecans
Peppers (red and green)
Potatoes (new, small)
Spring onions
Strawberries

Snack	Dinner	Snack
Laughing Cow Light cheese with high-fibre crispbread	Salmon Pasta (page 165)	Mixed berries tossed in lime juice with soured cream
Hummus with carrot and celery sticks	Pan-Seared White Fish with Mandarin Salsa (page 169), broccoli and basmati rice	Orange and almonds
Cottage cheese (low fat) with fruit slices	Chicken Schnitzel (page 171), green beans, carrots and new potatoes	Slice of Strawberry Tea Bread (page 184) and a glass of skimmed milk
Crunchy Chickpeas (page 181)	Mushroom and Gravy Pork Chops (page 179), asparagus and basmati rice	½ food bar
Laughing Cow Light cheese with high-fibre crispbread	Horseradish Burgers (page 176) and Tabbouleh Salad (page 156)	Mixed berries tossed in lime juice with soured cream
Hummus with carrot and celery sticks	Vegetarian Moussaka (page 164) and basmati rice	Slice of Strawberry Tea Bread (page 184) and a glass of skimmed milk
Fruit Yoghurt	Spicy Roasted Chicken with Tomatoes and Tarragon (page 174), green beans and basmati rice	Slice of One-Bowl Chocolate Cake (page 188) with berries

Sunflower seeds, shelled and unsalted
Tomatoes (large beefsteak, plum, and cherry or grape)
Tomatoes (sun-dried)
Walnuts

Deli
Feta cheese (light)
Hummus (light)
Lean deli ham
Lean deli turkey
Light herb and garlic cream cheese
Parmesan cheese, grated

Bakery
High-fibre crispbread
100% stone-ground wholemeal

bread
Wholemeal breadcrumbs
Wholemeal hamburger buns
Wholemeal pitta bread

Fish
Frozen crab
Salmon fillet
White fish fillets

Meat
Back bacon
Beef mince (extra-lean)
Boneless pork loin chops
Chicken breasts (boneless, skinless)

Beans (legumes) and tinned vegetables
Chickpeas
Kidney beans (red)
Lentils
Tomatoes (diced)
Tomatoes (plum)
Tomato puree

Pasta and sauces
Macaroni (wholemeal)
Small-shaped pasta (ditali or tubetti)

Soup and tinned seafood and meat
Chicken stock (low fat, low salt)

Grains and side dishes
Basmati rice
Bulgur wheat

International foods
Rice vinegar

Cooking oil, vinegar, salad dressings and pickles
Buttermilk salad dressing (low fat, low sugar)
Cooking oil spray (vegetable or olive oil)
Dijon mustard
Horseradish
Mayonnaise (fat-free)
Oil (vegetable and extra-virgin olive)
Red wine vinegar
Steak sauce
Wholegrain mustard
Worcestershire sauce

Snacks
Apple sauce (unsweetened)
Food bars (e.g. Slim-Fast)
Tinned mandarin oranges (no added sugar)

Baking
Baking powder
Bicarbonate of soda
Oat bran
Spices (ground allspice, dried basil, black pepper, cayenne pepper, ground cinnamon, ground cumin, Italian herb seasoning, nutmeg, oregano, red-pepper flakes, salt, dried thyme)
Splenda
Unsweetened cocoa powder
Vanilla extract
Wheat bran
Wheat germ
Wholemeal flour

Breakfast foods
All-Bran cereal
Oatmeal (large-flake oats)

Beverages
Apple juice (unsweetened)
Dry white wine (or vermouth)

Dairy
Buttermilk
Cottage cheese (low fat)
Fruit yoghurt (non-fat with sweetener)
Laughing Cow cheese (light)
Margarine (soft, non-hydrogenated, light)
Milk (skimmed)
Orange juice (unsweetened)
Soured cream (low fat)

Frozen foods
Mixed berries
Peas (or fresh)

Week 13 When Weight Loss Causes Anxiety

I would like to talk about the influence of social factors on the weight-loss experience. Many e-Clinic participants told me that they didn't want their family, friends and co-workers to know that they were trying to lose weight.

'I have not told any co-workers and only two close friends about being on the programme because of the fear of the "I told you so," "I knew you'd never stick to it," and "You're on another diet?" responses I have heard all my life from my mother and others ... Social situations are still uncomfortable for me and I am very self conscious of how I look.' – Kathy

'In group situations (especially with family) if I'm not eating what other people are eating, then people are going to talk. They're going to start asking me if I'm on a diet and I don't want to admit that I am, because my low self-esteem says that I'm not going to be able to do it, and then everyone will talk about what a failure I am.' – Lynette

'I often feel self-conscious because of my size and appearance so what better way to bury these bad feelings than with my old friend and comfort blanket: lots of food? Also I avoid calling attention to myself by reverting to old eating patterns so no one asks why I'm not overeating as usual, in other words acting normal to avoid scrutiny.' – Ross

Anxiety about being caught failing and feeling humiliated can be exacerbated when people start noticing your weight loss and ask questions like, 'Have you lost some weight?' or, 'What diet are you trying now?' You might start to feel as if you're being watched, and that people are wondering how long it will be before you give up. This is especially true if you have been a yo-yo dieter. The best defence in this case is to have a set of responses ready for their comments:

'Thank you for noticing.'

'Thanks. I'm going to need your support as I do this. Let me tell you how you can help ...'

'I know you want me to succeed, so I can improve my health. Let me tell you how you can help ...'

Family members can be the most discouraging. Here is an example:

'When my sister met me to drive me home, she commented on how she could tell that I had lost a significant amount of weight. That made me feel great. I said, "Oh, that reminds me that I have some dress pants that are getting too big." Her response was, "Oh, just put them in a box – you never know when you will need them again." Horrified, I said I would never need them again. How is that for a little encouragement and discouragement all at the same time?'

If you become the target of dispiriting comments like, 'So what's the magic diet this time round?' or 'How long will the weight be off this time?' try squelching them with kindness. Say something like, 'Jim, I'm sure you want me to succeed, so saying something supportive would be much more helpful.' Then smile – you'll feel better for taking the high road.

There can be some hidden anxiety about changing your body. Strange though it may seem when your greatest wish is to be slim and trim, deep down you may worry that you won't recognise the new you and that you won't be the same person.

Does personality change when you lose weight? Certainly, you may feel healthier, have more energy, sleep better, worry less and feel less depressed, but none of this has anything to do with your personality, which is formed early on and makes you unique and different from everyone else. Your personality is essentially who you are, and it's not going to change when you lose weight. If you have a wicked sense of humour, it's not going to disappear when you lose seven stone. If you are shy, losing weight isn't going to turn you into a party animal. You may feel more comfortable in social situations but you will still be you. Some of the defensive behaviours you developed to survive being large in the world may disappear with the pounds, but the fundamental you will remain. Excess weight is often subconsciously used to hide and protect the body. Ironically, being large can make people 'invisible', that is unnoticed or ignored.

Excess weight can be a way to de-sexualise the body, in that men and women can lose their sexual attractiveness and gender-specific qualities. We know from research that women with eating disorders such as anorexia sometimes use starvation to lose all their female sexual characteristics. Large women may similarly be hiding theirs with fat. The reasons can be complex. Some women with histories of sexual abuse do this as a means of protection, believing that men will not be attracted to a large asexual body. Losing excess weight can give the body a defined shape, making women look more feminine and men more masculine. They may suddenly be seen and noticed, and considered physically attractive or 'sexy', which may be anxiety producing. But the reality is that it is a whole lot easier living in this society when your body is not overweight. Slender people tend to be treated better than overweight people, and research shows that slender people are regarded as being brighter, richer and happier than those who are overweight. People who are attractive advance more quickly in the workplace.

Once you've lost a significant amount of weight and bought yourself a new wardrobe, start practising how you will behave in potentially anxiety-provoking situations. E-Clinic participants wrote me about some awkward situations:

'When people comment on my changing appearance ... it is sometimes difficult to suppress that inner voice that tends to "over think" things, and this leads to misinterpretation of a simple compliment. There are undeniable emotionally laden aspects to this process that lead to veering off the path, so to speak.'
– Bernadette

'So many people in my office have now bought your book (I bet at least nine people) and come to me regularly for help and guidance. It is so funny. They are all amazed at the physical transition. I wore low-waisted jeans last week and felt like a monkey in a zoo. People were coming by to look at me because someone else would say, "Have you seen Bev today? She looks great." I found it a little embarrassing. I kept apologizing and saying, "Well, I still have a lot to lose." My girlfriend told me to accept it and just say thanks because I've worked hard and it shows. (She is a big support).' – Beverley

Try to do some role-playing with a close friend. Have him or her comment on how good you look, pay you compliments, ask you out – whatever you might find difficult – and practise your responses. If someone comments on how good you look or likes your new outfit, practise looking them straight in the eye and saying thank you – no qualifying statements please! In our politically correct world it is unlikely anyone would dare tell you that you look 'sexy', but if they do, figure out what light comment you could make before contemplating filing a complaint!

As you start to make friends with and become familiar with your new body, remember that virtually everyone is dissatisfied with their bodies – even those whose bodies seem perfect. They too are filled with self-doubt and look for that new lotion or potion that will improve how they look. Where would the beauty industry be without all our anxieties? So don't think you're the only one worrying while everyone else feels secure about themselves. We all wish we could be better somehow. Just enjoy your lighter body, and remember that the goal is not perfection, but a more comfortable and healthy self.

Well, dear reader, by now you have completed a three-month journey on the Gi Diet. Some of you may have reached your target weight, while others will still have some way to go. In the next chapter, I will reveal the results achieved by some of our e-Clinic participants and include their thoughts on the programme.

Week 13 Weight ⬜ Week 13 Waist ⬜ Week 13 Hips ⬜

Week 13 Diary

_____
_____
_____
_____
_____
_____
_____
_____
_____

Optional week 13 meal plan

	Breakfast	Snack	Lunch
Mon	Homey Porridge (page 145) with chopped apple	Cranberry Cinnamon Bran Muffin (page 181)	Open-face chicken sandwich with lettuce, tomato and onion, and Basic Gi Salad (page 153)
Tue	Mini Breakfast Puffs (page 147)	Fruit yoghurt	Gi Pasta Salad (page 156)
Wed	Homemade Muesli (page 145) with skimmed milk and fruit yoghurt	Cranberry Cinnamon Bran Muffin (page 181)	½ wholemeal pitta with tuna, lettuce, tomato and cucumber, and Basic Gi Salad (page 153)
Thu	Homey Porridge (page 145) with blueberries	Small apple and a glass of skimmed milk	Quick and Easy Chicken Noodle Soup (page 151) and Basic Gi Salad (page 153)
Fri	All-Bran with skimmed milk, peach slices and sliced almonds	Fruit yoghurt	Mixed Bean Salad (page 157)
Sat	Western Omelette (page 149)	½ food bar	Greek Salad (page 155)
Sun	Oatmeal Buttermilk Pancakes with Strawberries (page 146)	Orange and almonds	Tuscan White Bean Soup (page 151) and Basic Gi Salad (page 153)

Snack	Dinner	Snack
Laughing Cow Light cheese with high-fibre crispbread	Easy-Bake Lasagne (page 163) and Caesar Salad (page 154)	Mixed berries tossed in lime juice with soured cream
Hummus with carrot and celery sticks	Gi Fish Fillet (page 166), asparagus, carrots and new potatoes	Orange and almonds
Fruit yoghurt	Chicken Curry (page 170) and Raita Salad (page 152)	Apple Pie Cookie (page 188) and a glass of skimmed milk
Crunchy Chickpeas (page 181)	Vegetable Crumble (page 161) and Tabbouleh Salad (page 156)	$^3/_4$ food bar
Laughing Cow Light cheese with high-fibre crispbread	Chicken Fried Rice (page 170)	Mixed berries tossed in lime juice with soured cream
Hummus with carrot and celery sticks	Beef and Aubergine Chilli (page 176) and Basic Gi Salad (page 153)	Apple Pie Cookie (page 188) and a glass of skimmed milk
Fruit yoghurt	Pork Medallions Dijon (page 178), green beans, carrots and new potatoes	Piece of Plum Crumble (page 186)

Week 13 shopping list for meal plan

Produce
Almonds (whole and sliced)
Apples
Asparagus
Aubergines
Baby spinach
Bean sprouts
Blueberries or mixed summer berries
(fresh or frozen)
Broccoli
Carrots
Celery
Courgettes
Cranberries (dried)
Cucumbers
Fresh herbs (chives, mint, flat-leaf
parsley, sage, tarragon, thyme)
Garlic
Green beans
Kale
Leeks
Lemons
Lettuce (iceberg, leaf and Cos)
Mixed nuts
Mushrooms
Onions (yellow and red)
Oranges
Peaches (fresh or canned in juice or
water)
Peppers (red and green)
Plums
Potatoes (new, small)
Raisins
Sesame seeds
Spring onions
Strawberries
Sunflower seeds (shelled, unsalted)
Sweet potato
Tofu (firm)
Tomatoes (plum)

Deli
Feta cheese (light)

Hummus (light)
Kalamata olives
Parmesan cheese

Bakery
High-fibre crispbread
100% stone-ground wholemeal
bread
Wholemeal pitta bread

Fish
Fish fillets (salmon or trout)

Meat
Back bacon
Beef mince (extra-lean)
Chicken breasts (boneless, skinless)
Pork tenderloins

Beans (legumes) and tinned vegetables
Chickpeas
Kidney beans (red and white)
Mixed beans
Tomatoes (diced)
Tomatoes (plum)
Tomato puree

Pasta and sauces
Fusilli or penne (wholemeal)
Small-shaped pasta (e.g. ditali or
tubetti)
Lasagne (wholemeal)
Light tomato sauce (no added sugar)
Low-fat pasta sauce (no cheese or
meat in sauce)

Soup and tinned seafood and meat
Anchovy fillets
Chicken stock (low fat, low salt)
Tuna (light, in water)
Vegetable stock (low fat, low salt)

Grains and side dishes
Basmati rice
Brown rice
Bulgur wheat
Flaxseeds (ground)

International foods
Sesame oil
Soy sauce (low sodium)
Tahini

Cooking oil, vinegar, salad dressings and pickles
Cooking oil spray (vegetable or olive oil)
Dijon mustard
Mayonnaise (fat-free)
Oil (vegetable and extra-virgin olive)
Red wine vinegar
Worcestershire sauce

Snacks
Apple sauce (unsweetened)
Food bars (e.g. Slim-fast)

Baking
Baking powder
Bicarbonate of soda
Cornflour
Oat bran
Spices (ground cardamom, cayenne, chilli powder, ground cinnamon, ground cumin, curry powder, ground ginger, ground nutmeg, dried oregano, black pepper, red-pepper flakes, salt, dried thyme)

Splenda
Vanilla extract
Wheat bran
Wheat germ
Wholemeal flour

Breakfast foods
All-Bran cereal
Oatmeal (large-flake oats)

Beverages
White wine

Dairy
Buttermilk
Cheddar cheese (low fat)
Cottage cheese (low fat)
Fruit yoghurt (non-fat with sweet-ener)
Laughing Cow cheese (light)
Margarine (soft, non-hydrogenated, light)
Milk (skimmed)
Mozzarella cheese (low fat)
Plain yoghurt (non-fat)
Soured cream (light)
Whole omega-3 eggs

Frozen foods
Mixed berries
Peas (or fresh)

5

Results of the e-Clinic

I'm sure you're all wondering how everyone did after the first thirteen weeks of the e-Clinic. Well, I'm really delighted with the participants' overall progress. I'm happy to report that we had a dropout rate of less than 20 per cent – and that includes those who had to leave the programme for medical reasons, such as chemotherapy and hip replacement. Those who stayed with it lost significant amounts of weight. In this chapter, I will share with you the results of some of the participants as well as their comments about what they learned and experienced while on the programme. Now of course the results varied from person to person, but this is in no way a reflection of their commitment or of their achievements – we all have different body shapes, metabolisms, ages and medical histories and we all lose weight at different rates. They all deserve a big pat on the back!

From Bernadette, who lost one and a half stone and a total of eight inches from her waist and hips:

'I can honestly say that I never felt hungry or deprived during the thirteen weeks. This is probably the most significant and critical difference from other weight-loss approaches that I have tried. Not having to measure and weigh most of the food that I eat has probably been the next most critical factor in the success that I have experienced to date. Having to do that in the past with other weight-loss programmes and then keep track of points was not compatible with real life and quickly gave way to resentment and failure.

I do like that the range of choices is so broad in most categories of foods listed and that you don't have a feeling of restriction ... I believe that the difference between success at this process of weight loss and failure is quickly overcoming a setback, whether it be making a bad choice or however you want to describe not sticking to the plan. I have come to understand that putting a setback behind you and getting quickly back on track is the key to success. Anything else just perpetuates that "I blew it and what's the point" feeling and holds you back ... I appreciate your support and I am excited about the continued feeling of vitality that I have rediscovered. For that I am very grateful.'

From Diane, who lost almost one and a half stone:

'I am still a little disappointed with my total lost amount but I know that I am

down below what I have been for the past seven years. That is encouraging and I know I will continue the good eating habits I have practiced the last three months ... I think that my husband and I have always practiced pretty good "home cooking" eating habits – we already used low-fat, sugar-free items and ate lean meats. But I have had a big problem with being a "stress eater" and a "social eater" (going out to restaurants, inviting people over, fast food convenience). You have helped me with these issues a lot! Having items for snacks has greatly helped! ... I have so much more energy this season than I did a year ago. I can remember last year I didn't even want to put up my Christmas decorations because I just did not have the energy. This year I feel back to my old self. Now I just need to find that self that I haven't seen since around 1995 (when I was diagnosed with asthma and started gaining my weight back)! I know I can do this – for me!

Thanks again! It has been a great three months!'

From Ross, who lost over three stone:

'One of the biggest obstacles I personally have found, besides all the usual ones, is poor planning as far as shopping goes. I would run out of green-light items and occasionally revert "just this once" to red-light foods as they were now quicker because "I didn't have time to go shopping at the moment and needed to eat." I now work out a plan for a week or so, listing the days and the meals and a possible "menu" ... This only takes a few minutes to actually do the "maths" and write the list, plus of course I have to actually get the shopping done.'

From Karen, who lost over a stone and a total of 7 inches from her waist and hips:

'My biggest suggestion for others is to have as much green-light food around you as possible for the situations you can control. I can control my home and my office (meaning my immediate office, not the communal kitchen). I cannot control what is available when I am at other people's homes or the office cafeteria, which still serves meatloaf and mashed potatoes or pizza as your two hot choices! I can (however dorky it seems) bring two slices of high-fibre wholemeal bread in my purse, get the insides of my sandwich from the salad bar and make my own sandwich at the table. Restaurants take practice, but as you've said there are usually enough good choices to cobble together a meal. I've eaten out an average of three lunches and three dinners per week and still have lost weight. Of course the weeks I brown bag it and eat dinner at home I have better results.

I've also learned that I share my home and office with "diet assassins". I think they think if they can get me to cheat, it absolves their bad eating habits. Last night I found myself making chocolate-chip cookies because my husband and co-workers requested them because "[mine] are the best ever". As I was dropping the dough on to the cookie sheet I had an epiphany. I told my husband he could bake as many as he wanted and I wrapped up the rest of the raw dough and brought it in to my co-workers with baking instructions. You go, girl!

The hardest thing has been adjusting expectations as the weeks wore on. The first few weeks the weight dropped right off me. I was taking the initial weight loss, multiplying by the number of weeks until New Year's Eve, and eyeing a new cocktail dress. No such luck. Things ground to a halt after the eighth or ninth week, with only modest losses. But, I'm still down over a stone and have either lost a minimal amount or not gained during the holiday season ... Rick, thank you for choosing me to be in the group and for your and Ruth's tremendous support during this part of the voyage.'

From Kathy, who lost two stone and a total of 19 inches from her waist and hips:

'What have I learned over the past thirteen weeks? An enormous amount about myself: that I can say no and mean it, that I can socialise and do okay, that having someone else to share the journey with makes all the difference in the world, that it feels good to accomplish something and see the results beginning to change your thinking and actions, that there is a lot of bad information there is out there about food and diet that I spent years following and being frustrated with, that I don't have to be hungry or feel like I am being deprived, that I look forward to the weekly weigh-in with positive anticipation rather than negative fear, that whatever happened in childhood is no excuse for being overweight now – what's done is done, forget it, move on! Thank you for opening my eyes to all of this and my mind to accepting it.'

From Pat, who lost over a stone:

'I am proud of myself this week as I have not only lost more inches, but I am down another pound ... What really matters is the weight continues to drop and I am bound and determined to reach my goal of ten stone ... As for what tips I can provide, I always ask myself when I think I'm starving, "Am I hungry, thirsty or tired?" Also when I am really wanting those red-light foods, I say to myself, "Do I really need them or want them?" This gets me back on track. I also think about the end result and how I will look and feel. I know that summer is only months away and I want to look fine.

When people comment on my weight loss and ask what diet I am on, I inform them this is my new way of eating. I have changed my lifestyle to improve my overall health ... I keep using the red leather jacket as motivation. I try it on every Sunday morning to see the progress I have made and it helps me to stay motivated.'

From Nancy, who lost almost a stone and over 10 inches from her waist and hips:

'Gosh, sometimes this is such a mental struggle! Like many people, I've used food as a source of comfort over the years, particularly sweets. I spent two days in the hospital this week (asthma), so I felt sorry for myself and let myself eat things I know better than to eat – what's up with that? It's so frustrating.

I think it's a mindset thing, in that I need to get back to the place where I simply choose not to eat sweets, where it's not even an option, let alone a desire. Does that make sense? I've reached that place with fried foods, in that I physically cannot handle eating anything fried anymore. I want to reach that same place with sweets, though admittedly they've had a much stronger "hold" over me than fried foods ever did.

Ah well, it's a journey and I press on. Besides, I have to remember that not only am I working towards losing weight and regaining my physical health, but I'm also sorting through a lot of long-standing mental attitudes at the same time. It's all part of the long-term success, I think, in that I have to deal with all aspects of the weight gain, not just the physical.'

Congratulations everyone!

Where to go from here

Whether you have reached your weight-loss target by now, and are ready to start Phase II of the Gi Diet (see Chapter 6), or still have some way to go, I would like to offer you what the original e-Clinic participants were offered at the end of the first 13 weeks of the e-Clinic: a nine-month extension of the programme which includes a monthly e-letter. These monthly e-letters will cover issues such as:

- How to stay the course
- Anxiety and fear of failure
- Maintaining motivation
- Dealing with temptation
- 5 essentials to permanent weight loss

The original e-Clinic members, whether they wished to maintain their weight or still had more weight to lose, found this extension of the basic 13-week programme extremely valuable. If you'd like to receive these nine monthly e-mail letters and record your progress on an optional personal website diary, all you have to do is to register at www.gidietclinic.com.

An exclusive website will support you during these nine months through a special members question and answer forum, where I will respond to major issues raised in participants' diaries. In addition you will receive access to recipes not available anywhere else online.

Once you register at www.gidietclinic.com, you will receive the first letter immediately as well as access to your personal diary should you wish to track your results. All your personal information will be kept strictly confidential. Any use of your questions or comments on the website will refer only to your first name.

The e-Clinic is a great opportunity to continue your positive experience with the Gi Diet.

For those of you who do not intend to continue with the nine-month extension, I would be most grateful if you would forward to me your weekly results from the 13 weeks in this book. If this is too much trouble, then just send me your starting measurements and your Week 13 measurements. Simply go to www.gidietclinic.com and click on the link to submit your results through a simple form. Any comments you might have would also be greatly appreciated.

6

Phase II

Well, you've made it. Congratulations! You've hit your target weight, you're digging out clothes you thought you'd never get into again, and you're finally on good terms with your full-length mirror. I hope you are relishing the new you and making the most of your increased energy. Now that you've graduated from Phase I, you can ease up a bit on limiting portion and serving sizes, and start adding some yellow-light foods to your diet. The idea here is to get comfortable with your Gi programme; this is how you're going to eat for the rest of your life.

The best news for most of us in Phase II is about alcohol and chocolate. While both were considered red-light in the Preliminary Phase and Phase I because of their high calorie content and tendency to spike blood sugar levels, in Phase II it's time to reintroduce those little pleasures.

Alcohol

Medical research indicates that red wine, which is rich in flavonoids, can help reduce your risk of heart disease and stroke. So, in Phase II, a glass of red wine is allowed with dinner. Just because one glass is beneficial, however, doesn't mean that two or three are even better for you. Immoderate drinking undoes any health benefits, and alcohol contains calories. One glass of wine (5fl oz maximum) provides the optimum benefit.

Apart from red wine, keep your consumption of alcohol to a minimum. I realise that this can be difficult, since drinking is so often a part of social occasions and celebrations. An occasional lapse won't do a lot of harm, but it's easy to get carried away. There are various strategies to combat the social pressure to drink: you can graciously accept that glass of wine or cocktail, raise it in a toast, take a sip and then discreetly leave it on the nearest buffet table. Faced with a tray of vodka martinis and glasses of red wine, stick with the wine, which lasts longer. Ruth drinks spritzers (wine mixed with soda water) on special occasions. And if you add lots of ice to your spritzer, you can reduce the alcohol even further while still joining in the party spirit. Whatever strategy you choose, always try to eat some food with your drink, even if it has to be a forbidden piece of cheese. The fat will slow the absorption of the alcohol and minimise its impact. (Of course, better to gravitate to the vegetable tray, but an emergency canapé won't be the ruin of you.)

Chocolate

For many of us, living without chocolate is not living. The good news is that in Phase II some chocolate – the right sort of chocolate in the right amount – is acceptable. You may have heard that chocolate, like red wine, contains natural elements that help keep the arteries clear – but that's probably not your main motive for eating it. Chocolate combines fat, sugar and cocoa, all three of which please the palate. But most chocolate contains too much saturated fat and sugar, which keeps it deep in the red-light zone. Chocolate with a high cocoa content (70 per cent or more) delivers more chocolate intensity per ounce, which means that even a square or two is satisfying. A square or two can give chocoholics the fix they need.

Green-Light Servings

PHASE II

Chocolate (at least 70 per cent cocoa)	2 squares
Red wine	5fl oz glass (one)

Moderation is key

Phase II, I must warn you, is a bit of a danger zone, the stage when most diets go off the rails. Most people think that, when they reach their weight-loss goal, they can just drop the diet and go back to their old eating habits. And frankly, when I take a close look at what many of these diets expect you to live on, I can understand why people can't stick to them for long.

The reality is that, with some modifications, the Gi programme is your diet for life. But this shouldn't be a hardship, because the Gi Diet was designed to give you a huge range of healthy choices, so you won't feel hungry, bored or unsatisfied. By now, you will know how to navigate your green-light way through the supermarket, decipher food labels and cook the green-light way. You are likely to not even be tempted to revert to your old ways. If you should fall prey to a double cheeseburger, you will be dismayed at how heavy, sluggish and ungratified you feel afterward. You will be too attached to your new feeling of lightness and level of energy to abandon them.

Before we look at some of the new options open to you in Phase II, a word of caution: your body can now function on less food than it did before you started. Why? Because you're lighter now, and so your body requires fewer calories. Also, your metabolism has become more efficient, and your body has learned to do more with fewer calories. Keeping these two developments in mind, add a few more calories in Phase II, but don't go berserk. Don't make any significant changes in your serving sizes, and remember to make yellow-light foods the exception rather than the rule. This way you will keep the balance between the calories you're consuming and the calories you're expending – and that is the secret to maintaining your new weight.

As you modestly increase portions of foods that you particularly enjoy and include some yellow-light items as a treat, keep monitoring your weight weekly, and adjust your servings up or down until your weight stays stable. This may take a few weeks of experimentation, but when you've reached the magic balance and can stay there comfortably, that's the formula for the rest of your days.

Here are some ideas of how you might alter the way you eat in Phase II.

Breakfast

- Increase cereal serving size from 50g to 75g.
- Add a slice of 100% whole-grain toast and a pat of margarine.
- Double the amount of sliced almonds on your cereal.
- Enjoy an extra slice of back bacon.
- Have a glass of unsweetened juice now and then.
- Add one of the yellow-light fruits – a banana or apricot – to your cereal.
- Go caffeinated in the coffee department, if you like, but try to keep it to one cup a day.

Lunch

I suggest you continue to eat lunch as you did in Phase I, as this is the one meal that already contained some compromises in the weight-loss portion of the programme.

Dinner

- Add another boiled new potato.
- Increase the pasta serving from 40g to 60g uncooked.
- As a special treat, have a 170g (6oz) steak instead of a 110g (4oz) one.
- Eat a few more olives and nuts – but only a few!
- Try a cob of sweet corn with a dab of margarine.
- Add a slice of high-fibre bread or crispbread.
- Enjoy a yellow-light cut of lamb or pork.

Snacks

- Have a maximum of 1/3 packet of air-popped popcorn.
- Increase your serving size of nuts to 10 or 12.
- Enjoy a square or two of 70 per cent cocoa dark chocolate.
- Have a banana.
- Indulge in a scoop of low-fat ice cream or frozen yoghurt.

Of course, Phase II is not, and shouldn't be, a straitjacket. If you live 90 per cent within the guidelines of the diet, you are doing well. The idea that certain foods are completely and forever forbidden would drive you, sooner or later, back into their clutches. With the Gi Diet, you are in control of what you eat, and that includes (with discipline, moderation and common sense) almost everything.

TO SUM UP

1. In Phase II, use moderation and common sense in adjusting portions and servings.

2. Don't view Phase II as a straitjacket. Occasional lapses are fine.

The Recipes

All recipes sourced from Rick Gallop's Gi Diet series of books

BREAKFAST

HOMEY PORRIDGE (Makes 4 servings)

This hot breakfast is guaranteed to keep you feeling satisfied all morning. You can vary the flavour by topping it with fresh fruit such as berries or chopped apple.

500ml/18fl oz skimmed milk
350ml/12fl oz water
¾tsp cinnamon
½tsp salt

125g /4 ½oz large flake oats
4tbsp wheatgerm
25g/1oz chopped almonds
3tbsp Splenda

1. In a large pot, bring the milk, water, cinnamon and salt to boil. Stir in the oats and wheat germ and return to the boil. Reduce the heat to low and cook, stirring, for about 8 minutes or until thickened. Stir in the almonds and Splenda and serve.

HOMEMADE MUESLI (Makes 8–9 servings)

This cereal makes a delicious and healthy start to the day. Be sure to prepare it the night before so that it's ready to enjoy in the morning. Combine a serving of the Muesli with 5–6tbsp skimmed milk or water, cover and chill overnight. Then in the morning, stir in a 140g carton of fat and sugar free fruit yoghurt, or pop it in the microwave for a minute or so for a hot breakfast.

180g/6oz large flake oats
30g/1 ¼oz oat bran
75g/3oz sliced almonds
60g/2 ¼oz shelled unsalted
sunflower seeds

2tbsp wheatgerm
¼tsp cinnamon

1. In large re-sealable plastic food bag, combine all the ingredients together and press to seal tightly. Using a rolling pin, crush the mixture into coarse crumbs. Shake the bag to mix and store until required.

CINNAMON FRENCH TOAST (Makes 2 servings)

Serve this family favourite with slices of ham or back bacon and extra strawberries for a complete breakfast.

3 medium free range eggs
125ml/4 ½fl oz skimmed milk
1tbsp Splenda
1tsp vanilla extract
½tsp ground cinnamon
Pinch salt
4 slices stone-ground wholemeal bread
1tsp vegetable oil
100g/3 ½oz strawberries, sliced
1x140g carton fat and sugar free fruit yoghurt

1. In a shallow dish, whisk together the eggs, milk, Splenda, vanilla, cinnamon and salt. Dip each slice of bread into the egg mixture, making sure to coat both sides.

2. Meanwhile, brush the oil on to a non-stick griddle or large non-stick frying pan over a medium-high heat. Cook the dipped slices for about 4 minutes, turning once, or until golden brown. Serve with strawberries and yoghurt.

OATMEAL BUTTERMILK PANCAKES
(Makes 16 pancakes, 4 to 6 servings)

Make pancake breakfasts a weekend tradition. Serve them with fresh fruit or apple sauce.

70g/2½oz large flake oats
500ml/18fl oz buttermilk
160g/5 ½oz wholemeal flour
4tbsp ground flaxseed
1tbsp Splenda
1tsp ground cinnamon
1tsp bicarbonate of soda
1tsp baking powder
¼tsp salt
2 medium free range eggs
2tbsp vegetable oil
1tsp vanilla extract

1. In a bowl, soak the oats in buttermilk for 20 minutes.

2. In a large bowl, combine the flour, flaxseed, Splenda, cinnamon, bicarbonate, baking powder and salt.

3. In a third bowl, whisk together the eggs, oil and vanilla. Stir in the soaked oats and buttermilk. Pour over the flour mixture and stir until just mixed.

4. Meanwhile, heat a non-stick griddle or large non-stick frying pan over medium heat. Ladle a small ladle (about 4 tbsp) of batter on to the griddle for each pancake. Cook until bubbles appear on top, about 2 minutes.

5. Flip the pancakes and cook for another 1–2 minutes or until golden. Transfer to a plate and cover to keep warm. Repeat with remaining batter.

MINI BREAKFAST PUFFS (Makes 12 puffs, 6 to 8 servings)

Ideal for rushed mornings, these muffin-sized puffs are packed with nutrition.

1tsp vegetable oil
½ onion, diced
1 red pepper, seeded and diced
Broccoli florets from ½ head, roughly chopped
1 ½tsp fresh thyme
¼tsp each salt and freshly ground pepper
125g/4 ½oz light feta cheese, crumbled
6 medium free range eggs, beaten
250ml/9 fl oz skimmed milk
4tbsp wheat bran
4tbsp wholemeal flour

1. Preheat the oven to 200°C, Gas 6.

2. In a non-stick frying pan, heat the oil over a medium heat. Cook the onion and red pepper for about 5 minutes or until softened. Add the broccoli, thyme, salt and pepper; cover and steam for about 3 minutes or until the broccoli is just tender and bright green. Divide the mixture among 12 greased deep muffin tins.

3. Sprinkle the feta over the top of the vegetable mixture in each cup.

4. In a bowl, whisk together the eggs, milk, bran and flour. Divide evenly over the vegetable mixture. Bake for about 20 minutes or until golden, set and puffed. Let cool slightly before serving.

BACK BACON OMELETTE (Makes 1 serving)

The smoky flavour of bacon makes this omelette a hit. Serve this with fresh fruit and yoghurt for a hearty breakfast.

1tsp vegetable oil
2 medium free range eggs
1tbsp chopped fresh basil
1tbsp grated Parmesan cheese
Pinch freshly ground pepper
2 slices back bacon or ham, chopped
¼ red or green pepper, chopped

1. In a small non-stick frying pan heat the oil over a medium-high heat. In a bowl, using a fork, stir together the eggs, basil, cheese and pepper. Pour into the frying pan and cook for about 5 minutes, lifting the edges to allow the uncooked egg to run underneath, until almost set.

2. Sprinkle the bacon and red or green pepper over half of the omelette. Using a spatula, fold over the other half and cook for 1 minute.

ITALIAN OMELETTE (Makes 1 serving)

Omelettes are easy to make, and you can vary them by adding any number of fresh vegetables, a little cheese and/or some meat.

1tsp vegetable oil
125g/4 ½oz mushrooms, sliced
2 medium free range eggs
1x140g can tomato purée
1tbsp chopped fresh basil or oregano
25g/1oz grated reduced-fat mozzarella cheese
Pinch freshly ground pepper

1. In a small non-stick frying pan heat the oil over medium-high heat. Add the mushrooms and sauté until tender, about 5 minutes. Transfer the mushrooms to a plate and cover to keep warm.

2. In a bowl, using a fork, stir together the eggs, tomato purée, basil, cheese and pepper. Pour into the frying pan and cook for about 5 minutes, lifting the edges to allow the uncooked egg to run underneath, until almost set.

3. Sprinkle the sautéed mushrooms over half of the omelette. Using a spatula, fold over the other half and cook for 1 minute.

VEGETARIAN OMELETTE (Makes 1 serving)

1tsp vegetable oil
Florets from ½ head broccoli
125g/4 ½oz mushrooms
4tbsp each chopped red and green pepper
2 medium free range eggs
25g/1oz grated reduced-fat Cheddar
Pinch freshly ground pepper

1. In a small non-stick frying pan heat the oil over a medium-high heat. Add the broccoli, mushrooms and pepper and sauté until tender, about 5 minutes.

Transfer the vegetables to a plate and cover to keep warm.

2. In a bowl, using a fork, stir together the eggs, cheese and pepper. Pour into the frying pan and cook for about 5 minutes, lifting the edges to allow the uncooked egg to run underneath, until almost set.

3. Sprinkle sautéed vegetables over half of the omelette. Using a spatula, fold over the other half and cook for 1 minute.

WESTERN OMELETTE (Makes 1 serving)

1tsp vegetable oil
½ red pepper, chopped
½ green pepper, chopped
1 small onion, chopped
2 medium free range eggs
2 slices lean back bacon, chopped
Pinch red pepper or chilli flakes or cayenne pepper

1. In a small non-stick frying pan heat the oil over a medium-high heat. Add the peppers and onions, and sauté until tender, about 5 minutes. Transfer the vegetables to a plate and cover to keep warm.

2. In a bowl, using a fork, stir together the egg, bacon and red pepper or chilli flakes. Pour into the frying pan and cook for about 5 minutes, lifting the edges to allow the uncooked egg to run underneath, until almost set.

3. Sprinkle the sautéed vegetables over half of the omelette. Using a spatula, fold over the other half and cook for 1 minute.

SOUPS

MINESTRONE SOUP (Makes 6 servings)

This soup is one of my favourites because it contains both pasta and spinach. Serve it with a sprinkling of grated Parmesan cheese for extra flavour and a few more red pepper flakes to get your blood pumping.

2tsp vegetable oil
3 slices back bacon, chopped
1 onion, chopped
4 cloves garlic, crushed
2 carrots, chopped
1 stick celery, chopped
1tbsp dried oregano
½tsp red pepper or chilli flakes or to taste
¼tsp each salt and freshly ground pepper
1×400g can chopped plum tomatoes
1.5 litres/2 ¾ pints chicken stock, made with a cube
1×225g bag baby leaf spinach
1×410g can red kidney beans, drained and rinsed
1×410g can chickpeas, drained and rinsed
120g/4oz small pasta shapes or macaroni
6tbsp chopped fresh flat-leaf parsley
2tbsp chopped fresh basil (optional)

1. In a large soup pot heat the oil over a medium-high heat and cook bacon for 2 minutes. Reduce the heat to medium and add the onion, garlic, carrots, celery, oregano, red pepper or chilli flakes, salt and pepper. Cook for about 10 minutes or until the vegetables are softened and lightly browned.

2. Add the tomatoes and crush using a potato masher in the pot. Pour in the chicken stock and bring to boil. Reduce the heat to a simmer and add the spinach, beans, chickpeas and pasta. Simmer for about 20 minutes or until the pasta is tender. Stir in the parsley and basil (if using).

Vegetarian variation: Omit the back bacon and substitute vegetable stock for the chicken stock.

TUSCAN WHITE BEAN SOUP (Makes 4 servings)

Serve this soup in deep Italian ceramic soup bowls and dream you're in Tuscany.

1tbsp extra virgin olive oil
1 onion, chopped
4 cloves garlic, crushed
1 carrot, chopped
1 stick celery, chopped
4 fresh sage leaves or 1/2 tsp dried
1.5 litres/2 ¾ pints vegetable or chicken stock, made with a cube
2x410g cans cannellini or white kidney beans, drained and rinsed
320g/10 ½oz kale or dark green cabbage, shredded
Pinch freshly ground pepper

1. In a soup pot heat the oil over a medium heat. Add the onion, garlic, carrot, celery and sage and cook for 5 minutes or until softened.

2. Add the stock, beans and pepper, and cook, stirring occasionally, for about 10 minutes, then add kale and continue cooking 10 minutes until kale is tender.

QUICK AND EASY CHICKEN NOODLE SOUP
(Makes 6 servings)

Why buy canned soup when you can make this simple homemade version?

2tsp extra virgin olive oil
2 carrots, chopped
2 sticks celery, chopped
3 cloves garlic, chopped
1 onion, chopped
1tbsp chopped fresh thyme
1.5 litres/2 ¾ pints chicken stock, made with a cube
3 boneless skinless chicken breasts (125g/4 ½oz each), diced
200g/7oz frozen peas
60g/2 ¾ oz pasta shapes or macaroni
4tbsp chopped fresh flat-leaf parsley
¼tsp freshly ground pepper

1. In a large soup pot heat the oil over medium-high heat. Add the carrots, celery, garlic, onion and thyme, and cook for 10 minutes or until the vegetables are slightly softened.

2. Pour in the stock and bring to the boil. Reduce the heat to a simmer and add the chicken and pasta. Simmer for 10 minutes then add the peas and cook for another 5 minutes or until the chicken is no longer pink inside. Stir in the parsley and pepper.

HAM AND LENTIL SOUP (Makes 4 servings)

Canned lentils make this soup quick and easy to prepare, so keep some on hand. If you want to make this soup even more green-light, use dried lentils (see instructions at the bottom of this page).

1tbsp vegetable oil
1 onion, chopped
2 sticks celery, diced
2 cloves garlic, crushed
1.5 litres/2 ¾ pints chicken stock, made with a cube
2 x 410g cans lentils, drained and rinsed
180g/6oz lean deli ham, diced
1 red pepper, seeded and diced
2 tomatoes, seeded and diced
2tbsp chopped flat-leaf parsley

1. In a large soup pot heat the oil over a medium heat. Add the onion, celery and garlic and cook for about 5 minutes or until softened. Add the stock, lentils, ham and red pepper; bring to the boil. Reduce the heat and add the tomatoes. Cover and simmer for 20 minutes. Stir in the parsley.

Variation: Use 1 cup of dried green or brown lentils instead of canned. Mix in with the stock, cover and simmer for about 30 minutes or until tender.

SALADS

RAITA SALAD (Makes 4 servings)

This recipe is based on the refreshing Indian condiment. Try serving this salad with Chicken Curry (see recipe, page 170).

1x300g bag baby leaf spinach
½ cucumber, quartered lengthways and sliced into 1 cm/½ in chunks
2 tomatoes, chopped
½ red onion, thinly sliced
250g/9oz low-fat natural yoghurt
½tsp ground cumin
¼tsp salt

1. In a large bowl toss together the spinach, cucumber, tomatoes and red onion.

2. In another bowl stir together the yoghurt, cumin and salt. Toss into spinach mixture and serve.

TANGY RED AND GREEN COLESLAW
(Makes 4 to 6 servings)

Using a vinaigrette in coleslaw makes it low-fat and really tangy! This is a great salad to store for up to 2 days in the fridge to take along to a picnic or barbecue.

325g/10 ¹/₂oz finely shredded green cabbage
160g/5 ¹/₂oz finely shredded red cabbage
2 carrots, coarsely grated
2 sticks celery, thinly sliced
4tbsp chopped flat-leaf parsley

125ml/4 ¹/₂fl oz cider vinegar
2tbsp vegetable oil
2tsp Splenda
1tsp celery seeds
¹/₄tsp salt
Pinch freshly ground pepper

1. In a large bowl toss together the green and red cabbage, carrots, celery and parsley.

2. In a small bowl, whisk together the vinegar, oil, Splenda, celery seeds, salt and pepper. Pour over the cabbage mixture and toss to coat.

BASIC Gi SALAD (Makes 1 serving)

45g/1 ¹/₂ oz mixed leaf salad (e.g. Cos lettuce, rocket, baby leaf spinach or watercress), torn or coarsely chopped
1 small carrot, coarsely grated
¹/₂ red, yellow or green pepper, seeded and diced
1 plum tomato, cut into wedges
¹/₄ cucumber, sliced
¹/₂ small red onion, chopped (optional)

Basic Gi vinaigrette
1tbsp vinegar (such as balsamic, cider, red wine, rice or white wine) or lemon juice
1tsp extra-virgin olive oil or vegetable oil
¹/₂tsp Dijon mustard
1 clove garlic, crushed (optional)
Pinch each salt and freshly ground pepper
Pinch finely chopped fresh herb of choice (such as basil, marjoram, mint, oregano or thyme)

1. In a large bowl toss together the lettuce, carrot, pepper, tomato, cucumber and onion, if using.

2. In a small bowl whisk together the vinegar, oil, mustard, garlic, salt, pepper and herbs. Alternatively put all ingredients into a small screw-top jar, cover and shake to blend.

3. Pour the vinaigrette over vegetables and toss.

Variations: To make a meal out of this salad, add some protein with a 100g can of tuna, cooked salmon, tofu, kidney beans, chickpeas, cooked chicken or another lean meat.

CAESAR SALAD (Makes 4 servings)

A Caesar salad is a useful addition to your favourite recipe collection. In this special recipe, no one will guess that tahini is the secret ingredient that makes this green-light version every bit as creamy as a bought dressing.

3 slices wholemeal bread
2tsp extra virgin olive oil
Pinch each salt and freshly ground pepper
1 large head Cos lettuce
Dressing:
3 cloves garlic, crushed
3 anchovy fillets, finely chopped
2tbsp light tahini
1tsp Dijon mustard
½tsp Worcestershire sauce
½tsp each salt and freshly ground pepper
·3tbsp lemon juice
2tbsp warm water
1 ½tbsp extra virgin olive oil

1. Preheat the oven to 180°C, Gas 4.

2. Cut the bread into 1 cm/½ in pieces and place in a bowl. Add the oil, salt and pepper and toss to coat well. Arrange in a single layer in a shallow roasting tin. Bake for 20 minutes or until golden and crisp. Let cool.

3. Wash the lettuce and tear into bite-size pieces; place in a large bowl.

4. Make the dressing in a small bowl: stir together the garlic, anchovies, tahini, mustard, Worcestershire sauce, salt and pepper. Whisk in the lemon juice, water and oil.

5. Pour the dressing over lettuce and toss to coat. Sprinkle with croutons.

GREEK SALAD (Makes 2 servings)

About 100g/3½oz iceberg lettuce, torn
½ cucumber, chopped
2 tomatoes, chopped
6 Kalamata olives
½ red onion, sliced
4tbsp crumbled light feta cheese
1tbsp red wine vinegar
2tsp extra virgin olive oil
1tsp fresh lemon juice
¾tsp oregano
Pinch each of salt and freshly ground pepper

1. In a bowl toss together lettuce, cucumber, tomatoes, olives, red onion and feta.

2. In small bowl whisk together the vinegar, oil, lemon juice, oregano, salt and pepper. Pour the dressing over the lettuce and toss to coat.

COLD NOODLE SALAD WITH CUCUMBER AND SESAME (Makes 6 servings)

These refreshing noodles pair well with the Ginger-Wasabi Halibut (see recipe, page 167).

180g/6oz thin pasta (vermicelli or spaghettini)
1tbsp rice vinegar
4tsp Splenda
2tsp soy sauce
½ cucumber, quartered lengthwise and thinly sliced
2tbsp toasted sesame seeds

1. In a large pot of boiling salted water cook the pasta until al dente, about 4 minutes.

Drain and rinse under cold water. Place in a large bowl.

2. In a small bowl stir together the vinegar, Splenda and soy sauce. Pour over the cooked noodles, stir in the cucumber and sesame seeds; toss well to coat.

Gi PASTA SALAD (Makes 1 serving)

40g/1 ½oz wholemeal pasta (spirals, shells or similar shape)
100g/3 ½oz cooked vegetables (such as broccoli, asparagus, peppers or green onions)
4tbsp light tomato sauce or other low-fat or non-fat pasta sauce
125g/4 ½oz chopped cooked chicken

1. Cook the pasta, drain and allow to cool. Place the pasta, vegetables, tomato sauce and chicken in a bowl and stir to mix well. Cover and chill until ready to use, then serve chilled or heat it in the microwave to serve hot.

Variation: You can use the proportions here as a guide and vary the vegetables, sauce and source of protein to suit your tastes and add variety to your pasta salads.

TABBOULEH SALAD (Makes 4 to 6 servings)

You often see this salad in the grocery store deli, but it's very simple to make at home. The chickpeas add more fibre.

350ml/12fl oz water
120g/4oz bulgur
½tsp grated lemon zest
2tbsp lemon juice
2tbsp extra virgin olive oil
1 small clove garlic, crushed
½tsp each salt and freshly ground pepper
¼tsp ground cumin
1x410g can chickpeas, drained and rinsed
3 plum tomatoes, diced
¼ cucumber, diced
20g/¾oz finely chopped flat-leaf parsley
15g/½oz finely chopped fresh mint
1tbsp chopped fresh chives

1. In a saucepan bring water to boil; add bulgur. Cover, reduce heat to low and cook for about 10 minutes or until water is absorbed. Using fork, scoop into a large bowl and cool.

2. In a small bowl whisk together lemon zest and juice, oil, garlic, salt, pepper and cumin; pour over bulgur. Stir in chickpeas, tomatoes, cucumber, parsley, mint and chives and serve.

Make Ahead: This salad will last up to 3 days in the fridge.

MIXED BEAN SALAD (Makes 2 servings)

1x410g can mixed pulses, drained and rinsed
½ cucumber, chopped
1 tomato, chopped
180g/6oz cooked wholemeal pasta (small shells, macaroni or similar size)
2tbsp chopped fresh flat-leaf parsley
1tbsp red wine vinegar
2tsp extra virgin olive oil
¼tsp Dijon mustard
Pinch each of salt and freshly ground pepper
Pinch of fresh finely chopped herbs, such as thyme or oregano

1. Place the beans in a large bowl and add the cucumber, tomato, pasta and parsley.

2. In small bowl whisk together the vinegar, oil, mustard, salt, pepper and herbs.

Pour over the salad and toss to coat.

WALDORF CHICKEN AND RICE SALAD
(Makes 1 serving)

50g/1 ¾oz cooked basmati or brown rice
1 medium apple, chopped
1 stick celery, chopped
25g/1oz walnuts, roughly chopped
125g/4 ½oz cooked chicken, chopped
1tbsp reduced fat creamy dressing

1. Cook the rice and allow to cool. Place the rice, apple, celery, walnuts and chicken in a large bowl. Pour the dressing on top and stir to mix.

CRAB SALAD IN TOMATO SHELLS (Makes 4 servings)

Beefsteak tomatoes are ideal for this dish because their large size will accommodate the filling, and the pulp and seeds are easy to scoop out.

400g/14oz frozen white crabmeat, thawed
4 large beefsteak tomatoes
4tbsp fat free mayonnaise
2tbsp soured cream or reduced fat crème fraiche
½tsp grated lemon zest
1tbsp lemon juice
2tsp chopped fresh tarragon
Pinch each salt and freshly ground pepper
240g/8oz chopped cooked chickpeas
½ red pepper, diced
1 small stick celery, finely diced
4tbsp chopped flat-leaf parsley
2tbsp chopped fresh chives
2tbsp grated carrot

1. Place the crab in a fine-mesh sieve; press out any liquid with the back of a ladle. Tip out on to a large plate and, using a fork, check for any stray pieces of shell or cartilage if necessary; set aside the crab.

2. Cut the top quarter off the tomatoes. Using a small spoon, scoop out the seeds and pulp. Place the tomatoes, cut side down, on a paper-towel-lined plate.

3. In a large bowl stir together the mayonnaise, soured cream, lemon zest and juice, tarragon, salt and pepper. Add the chickpeas, red pepper, celery, parsley, chives and carrot, then stir in the crab. Spoon the mixture into the tomato shells.

Variation: Try using baby prawns, tuna or salmon instead of the crab.

MEATLESS

FETTUCCINE PRIMAVERA (Makes 4 servings)

Primavera means 'springtime' in Italian, and you can use your favourite spring vegetables, such as asparagus or courgettes, in this pasta. Fortunately, you can get peppers, tomatoes and peas year-round, so you can make this dish any time.

4tbsp extra virgin olive oil
320g/10 ¹/₂oz pack firm tofu, cubed
3 cloves garlic, crushed
¹/₄tsp red pepper or chilli flakes or to taste
125ml/4 ¹/₂fl oz vegetable cocktail juice
250g/9oz chopped fresh asparagus or peas
1 red pepper, seeded and thinly sliced
1 carrot, thinly sliced
1 courgette, yellow or green, thinly sliced
180g/6oz wholemeal fettuccine or linguine pasta
2 plum tomatoes, chopped
4tbsp chopped flat-leaf parsley
2tbsp grated Parmesan cheese

1. In a non-stick frying pan heat 2 tbsp of the oil over a medium-high heat. Brown the tofu on all sides for about 2 minutes; remove to a plate and drain into a large shallow saucepan. Add the remaining oil and heat.

2. Cook the garlic and red pepper flakes for 1 minute. Add the vegetable cocktail juice; bring to the boil. Reduce the heat and simmer for 1 minute. Add the asparagus, red pepper, carrot and courgette; cook, stirring, for 10 minutes or until the vegetables are just tender.

3. Meanwhile, in a large pot of boiling salted water cook the fettuccine for 8 minutes or until al dente. Drain and return to the pot. Add the vegetables and tofu, and toss to coat. Stir in the tomatoes, parsley and Parmesan cheese.

BARLEY RISOTTO WITH LEEKS, LEMON AND PEAS
(Makes 4 to 6 servings)

Unlike traditional risotto, this barley version doesn't need to be watched or stirred continuously.

1tbsp extra virgin olive oil
1 medium leek, chopped (white and light-green parts only)
2 cloves garlic, crushed
½tsp chopped fresh thyme
200g/7oz pearl barley
4tbsp dry white wine or vermouth
750 ml/1 ¼ pint chicken stock, made with a stock cube (and up to 150ml/¼ pint more if needed)
125g/4 ½oz fresh or thawed frozen peas
zest and juice 1 medium lemon
2tbsp grated Parmesan cheese
¼tsp each salt and freshly ground pepper

1. In a saucepan heat the oil over a medium-high heat; cook the leek, garlic and thyme, stirring, for 3 minutes or until softened. Stir in the barley until well coated.

2. Add the wine and stir until absorbed. Add the stock and bring to the boil. Cover and reduce the heat to low; simmer, stirring occasionally, for 40 to 45 minutes or until the barley is tender. If necessary, stir in a little more stock or hot water near the end of the cooking time to maintain a creamy consistency. Stir in the peas, lemon zest and juice and Parmesan cheese 5 minutes before the end of cooking; season with salt and pepper.

VEGETABLE CRUMBLE (Makes 4 to 6 servings)

We usually think of a crumble as dessert, but this one makes a delicious vegetarian main dish, or a side dish for meat or fish.

1tbsp extra virgin olive oil
1 large leek, sliced thinly (white and light-green parts only)
1 onion, chopped
1 courgette, cut into 2.5 cm/1 in pieces
1 large carrot, cut into 2.5 cm/1 in pieces
1 sweet potato, peeled and cut into 2.5cm/1 in pieces
125g/4¹⁄₂oz mushrooms, quartered
1 stick celery, sliced into 1 cm/¹⁄₂ in pieces
¹⁄₂ red pepper, seeded and cut into 2.5cm/1 in pieces
1tbsp chopped fresh thyme

4tbsp wholemeal flour
1x200g can plum tomatoes, roughly chopped
250ml/9fl oz vegetable stock, from a cube
125ml/4 ¹⁄₂fl oz skimmed milk
4tbsp chopped flat-leaf parsley
¹⁄₂tsp freshly ground pepper
Topping:
4tbsp soft margarine
4tbsp wholemeal flour
4tbsp wheat bran
75g/3oz grated reduced fat Cheddar cheese
150g/2oz chopped mixed nuts
2tbsp sesame seeds

1. Preheat the oven to 190°C, Gas 5.

2. In a large saucepan heat the oil over a medium-high heat. Cook the leeks and onion for 5 minutes or until softened. Add the courgette, carrot, sweet potato, mushrooms, celery, red pepper and thyme. Cook, stirring often, for 10 minutes. Stir in the flour; cook for 1 minute.

3. Stir in the tomatoes, stock, milk, parsley and pepper; bring to the boil. Reduce the heat, cover and simmer for about 15 minutes or until the vegetables are tender.

4. Topping: meanwhile in a bowl combine the margarine, flour and bran. Using your fingers, rub the ingredients together until the mixture is crumbly. Stir in the cheese, nuts and sesame seeds.

5. Spoon the vegetable mixture into a 2 litre/3 ¹⁄₂ pint shallow baking dish. Sprinkle the crumble mixture over the top, distributing evenly.

6. Bake for 30 minutes or until the topping is crisp and golden, and the vegetable mixture is bubbling.

Make Ahead: add 2tbsp wholemeal flour to filling in Step 2. After Step 5, wrap well and freeze up to 1 month. Bake from frozen, increasing cooking time by 30 to 45 minutes.

BEAN AND ONION PIZZA (Makes 4 servings)

Here's a restaurant favourite for your Gi lifestyle.

Pizza Dough:
160g/5 ¾oz wholemeal flour
20g/¾oz wheat bran
Pinch of salt
1 sachet fast action yeast
180ml/6fl oz warm water
Topping:
1tsp vegetable oil
2 onions, thinly sliced
2 cloves garlic, crushed
¾tsp finely chopped fresh thyme
Pinch each of salt and freshly ground pepper
4tbsp sun-dried tomatoes
120ml/4fl oz boiling water
150g/5oz cooked red kidney beans
½x350g jar pasta sauce
2tbsp chopped fresh basil
100g/3½oz crumbled light feta cheese

1. Pizza Dough: in a large bowl stir together the flour, bran, salt and yeast, then mix in the water to a ragged dough. Place the dough on a lightly floured surface and knead it, adding extra water in dribbles if necessary until it forms a soft, slightly sticky dough. Place in a greased bowl, cover and let rest until doubled in bulk, about 1 hour.

2. Topping: heat the oil in a non-stick frying pan over a medium-high heat. Add the onions and garlic and cook, stirring, until the onions start to become golden, about 3 minutes. Reduce the heat to medium and add the thyme, salt and pepper. Continue cooking, stirring occasionally, until the onions are soft and golden brown, about 15 minutes.

3. Meanwhile, soak the sun-dried tomatoes in the boiling water for 5 minutes. Drain and discard the water and chop the tomatoes.

4. Preheat the oven to 220°C, Gas 7.

5. Punch down the dough and roll it out on a floured surface to fit a 30–40 cm/12- or 14 in round pizza pan. Place the dough on the pan, stretching it as necessary to fit.

6. Put the beans in a large mixing bowl and mash them, using a potato masher. Stir in the pasta sauce, sun-dried tomatoes and basil. Spread the topping over the pizza dough. Top with the sautéed onions, and sprinkle with feta.

7. Bake for about 20 minutes or until golden and crisp.

EASY-BAKE LASAGNE (Makes 8 servings)

Though cooking the Gi way usually means starting from scratch, there are some handy convenience products that are green-light, such as pasta sauce! This lasagne is great for a crowd. Just add a tossed salad.

12 wholemeal lasagne sheets
2tsp vegetable oil
1 onion, chopped
1 red pepper, seeded and chopped
250g/9oz mushrooms, sliced
¼tsp each salt and freshly ground pepper
1x250g bag baby leaf spinach
240g/8oz diced firm tofu
1x250g tub low-fat cottage cheese
3 free range eggs, beaten
2x350g jars pasta sauce
150g/5oz reduced fat mozzarella cheese, grated
2tbsp grated Parmesan cheese

1. Preheat the oven to 180°C, Gas 4.

2. In a large pot of boiling salted water cook the lasagne sheets for about 10 minutes or until al dente. Drain and rinse under cold water. Lay the sheets flat on damp tea towels; set aside.

3. Meanwhile in a large non-stick frying pan heat the oil over a medium-high heat. Cook the onion, red pepper, mushrooms, salt and pepper for about 8 minutes, or until golden brown and softened. Add the spinach and cook, stirring, for 2 minutes or until wilted. Stir in the tofu.

4. In a small bowl stir together the cottage cheese and egg; set aside.

5. Spread a little of the pasta sauce in the bottom of a 23 x 32 cm/9 x 13-inch glass baking dish. Lay 3 pasta sheets on top of the sauce. Spread one third of the spinach mixture over the top then one third of the cottage cheese mixture. Spread with another layer of pasta sauce. Sprinkle with a handful of the mozzarella. Repeat layers, ending with sheets on top. Spread with the remaining sauce and sprinkle with the remaining mozzarella and Parmesan cheese. Cover with foil and bake for 45 minutes. Uncover and bake for 15 minutes until brown and a knife inserted in centre is hot to the touch. Let cool 10 minutes before cutting and serving.

VEGETARIAN MOUSSAKA (Makes 8 servings)

2 large aubergines,
about 650g/1 ½lbs each
2tsp salt
1tsp vegetable oil
2 large onions, finely chopped
3 cloves garlic, crushed
1 each red and green pepper, seeded
and diced
1tbsp dried oregano
1tsp ground cinnamon
½tsp freshly ground pepper
¼tsp ground allspice
2x400g cans chopped tomatoes
4tbsp tomato puree
1x400g can chickpeas, drained and
rinsed

4tbsp chopped fresh flat-leaf parsley
Cheese Sauce:
2tbsp vegetable oil
4tbsp wholemeal flour
500ml/18fl oz skimmed milk,
warmed
¼tsp salt
Pinch ground nutmeg
Pinch freshly ground pepper
4 free range eggs, beaten
125g/4 ½oz low-fat cottage cheese
125g/4 ½oz crumbled light feta
cheese

1. Preheat the oven to 220°C, Gas 7.

2. Cut the aubergines into 5mm/¼ inch thick slices and layer them in a colander, sprinkling each layer lightly with some of the salt. Let stand for 30 minutes, then rinse the slices and drain them well. Place them on baking sheets lined with non-stick baking parchment paper and roast, in batches if necessary, for about 20 minutes or until tender. Set aside. Reduce oven temperature to 180°C, Gas 4.

3. Heat the oil in a large, shallow Dutch oven or deep non-stick frying pan over a medium heat. Add the onions, garlic, red and green peppers, oregano, cinnamon, pepper and allspice, and cook until the onions have softened, about 5 minutes. Add the tomatoes and tomato puree and bring to a boil. Add the chickpeas and parsley, reduce the heat and simmer for 15 minutes.

3. Cheese Sauce: heat the oil in a saucepan over a medium heat. Stir in the flour and cook for 1 minute. Whisk in the milk and cook, whisking gently, for about 10 minutes or until the mixture is thick enough to coat the back of a spoon. Stir in the salt, nutmeg and pepper. Let cool slightly and whisk in the egg and cottage cheese.

4. Spread one third of the tomato sauce on the bottom of a 23 x 32cm/9 x 13in baking dish. Top with one third of the aubergine slices and one quarter of the feta cheese. Repeat the layers. After the last layer of aubergine, spread the cheese sauce evenly over the top and sprinkle with the remaining feta.

5. Bake for about 1 hour or until the top is golden brown. Let stand for 10 minutes before serving.

FISH AND SEAFOOD

SALMON PASTA (Makes 2 servings)

When you can't get fresh salmon, use 2 cans of salmon or tuna instead.

2tsp vegetable oil
1 small onion, finely chopped
2 cloves garlic, crushed
500ml/18fl oz chicken or fish stock, from a cube
115g/4oz macaroni
Florets from ½ head broccoli
85g/3oz light herb and garlic cream cheese
180g/6oz skinless salmon fillet
2tbsp chopped fresh flat-leaf parsley
Pinch each salt and freshly ground pepper

1. Preheat the oven to 220°C, Gas 7.

2. In a saucepan heat 1 tsp of the oil over a medium heat. Cook the onion and garlic for about 3 minutes or until softened. Add the chicken stock and bring to the boil. Add the pasta and cover; reduce the heat to a simmer and cook for 10 minutes. Stir in the broccoli and cream cheese. Remove from the heat. Let stand, covered, for 10 minutes while the salmon cooks.

3. Meanwhile, rub the remaining oil over the fillet and sprinkle with parsley, salt and pepper. Roast in a small baking pan for about 10 minutes or until the salmon is opaque and flakes easily with a fork. Break up the salmon into chunks and add to the pasta mixture. Stir gently to combine.

THAI RED CURRY PRAWN PASTA (Makes 4 servings)

Curry spices, lime and coriander are hallmarks of Thai cooking.

500g/1lb 2oz large raw tiger prawns, peeled and deveined
1tsp Thai red curry paste
1tbsp extra virgin olive oil
4 cloves garlic, crushed
2 large tomatoes, peeled, seeded and chopped
180ml/6oz dry white wine
Zest and juice of 1 lime
¼tsp each salt and freshly ground pepper
2tbsp chopped fresh coriander
180g/6oz wholemeal spaghetti
Lime wedges

1. In a bowl toss the prawns with the curry paste until well coated. Cover and chill for at least 2 hours and up to 8.

2. In a large non-stick frying pan heat the oil over a medium heat. Add the garlic and cook until just starting to turn golden, 1 to 2 minutes. Add the tomatoes, wine, lime zest and juice, and salt and pepper; bring to the boil, reduce the heat and simmer until the sauce reduces and thickens, about 8 minutes. Add the prawns and cook, stirring, until pink and firm, 3 to 4 minutes. Stir in the coriander.

3. Meanwhile, in a large pot of boiling salted water, cook the pasta until al dente, about 8 minutes. Drain and add the pasta to the prawn mixture. Toss to coat with the sauce. Serve with lime wedges.

Gi FISH FILLET (Makes 1 serving)

You can use virtually any fish in this simple recipe; salmon and trout are favourites in our house. This makes 1 serving, but you can multiply portions as necessary.

125g/4 ½ oz fish fillet
1 to 2tsp fresh lemon juice
Pinch freshly ground pepper

1. Place the fish fillet in a microwave-safe dish and sprinkle with lemon juice and a pinch of pepper. Cover the dish with microwave-safe plastic wrap, folding back one corner slightly to allow the steam to escape.

2. Microwave on high until the fish is opaque and flakes easily with a fork, 4 to 5 minutes. Let stand for 2 minutes, then serve.

CITRUS-POACHED HADDOCK (Makes 4 servings)

Citrus fruits and fish are made for each other. This simple dish is impressive enough for company.

1 small onion, finely chopped
1 clove garlic, crushed
4tbsp orange juice
4tbsp dry white wine or vermouth
1tbsp lemon juice
1tsp lemon zest
4tbsp fish, chicken or vegetable stock , made from a cube
500g/1lb 2oz haddock fillet, cut into 4 pieces
2tbsp chopped fresh flat-leaf parsley or dill
¼tsp freshly ground pepper

1. In a large frying pan bring the onion, garlic, orange juice, wine, lemon juice and zest to the boil. Boil until the onion is softened and the liquid is reduced by half, about 5 minutes.

2. Add the stock and return to the boil. Place the haddock in the frying pan; reduce the heat and simmer gently, covered, for 10 minutes or until the fish is opaque and flakes easily with a fork. Using a slotted spoon, remove the haddock to a platter and cover to keep warm.

3. Bring the poaching liquid to the boil and reduce by one third. Stir in the parsley and season with pepper. Pour the sauce over the fish.

GINGER-WASABI HALIBUT (Makes 4 servings)

This fish can also be cooked on the barbecue. Serve it with Cold Noodle Salad with Cucumber and Sesame (see recipe, page 155) for a refreshing meal.

2tbsp Dijon mustard
2tsp wasabi powder
3tbsp mirin or sweet sherry
2tbsp grated fresh root ginger
2tbsp chopped fresh coriander
500g/1lb 2oz halibut, cut into 4 pieces

1. In a bowl stir together the mustard and wasabi powder. Stir in the mirin, ginger and coriander. Place the fish in the marinade and turn to coat. Let stand at room temperature for 20 minutes.

2. Meanwhile, preheat the oven to 180°C, Gas 4. Place the halibut on a baking sheet and bake for 8 to 10 minutes or until firm to the touch.

GRILLED TUNA WITH CHIMICHURRI SAUCE
(Makes 4 servings)

Chimichurri is traditionally served with Argentinean barbecued beef (asado), but is also delicious with grilled tuna. This recipe makes extra sauce, which can be served with poultry or meat, or stirred into hot rice.

4 tuna steaks, about 1cm/1/2in thick
1/2tsp freshly ground pepper
Chimichurri Sauce:
4 cloves garlic, crushed
1/2 red onion, finely chopped
1/2 red pepper, seeded and finely chopped
4tbsp chopped fresh coriander
4tbsp chopped fresh flat-leaf parsley
1tbsp chopped fresh oregano
125ml/4 1/2oz vegetable stock, from a cube
2tbsp extra-virgin olive oil
2tbsp sherry or red wine vinegar
Pinch freshly ground pepper

1. Preheat an oiled grill to medium-high.

2. Chimichurri Sauce: in a bowl combine the garlic, red onion, red pepper, coriander, parsley and oregano. Stir in the stock, oil, sherry or vinegar and pepper.

3. Season the fish with pepper, and grill until just charred on outside and rare in centre, about 2 minutes per side. Serve with a dollop of Chimichurri Sauce on top.

Make Ahead: chill the sauce in an airtight container up to 5 days.

PAN-SEARED WHITE FISH WITH MANDARIN SALSA (Makes 4 servings)

A quick, bright, citrusy salsa lends a tropical note to this hearty fish fillet. You can use tilapia or haddock for this elegant meal.

Mandarin Salsa:
2x300g cans mandarin oranges in natural juice, drained
1 red pepper, seeded and diced
1/4 cucumber, finely diced
1/2 small red onion, finely diced
3tbsp chopped fresh coriander
1tbsp rice vinegar
1/4tsp salt
Pinch of freshly ground pepper
Fish Fillets:
50g/1 3/4oz fresh wholemeal breadcrumbs
4tbsp chopped fresh flat-leaf parsley
2tbsp wheat bran
2tbsp wheatgerm
1tbsp chopped fresh tarragon
1/4tsp salt
1/4tsp freshly ground pepper
4tbsp wholemeal flour
2 free range eggs, beaten
4 white fish fillets (125g/4 1/2oz each)
4tsp vegetable oil

1. Mandarin Salsa: coarsely chop the mandarin slices and place them in a bowl. Add the red pepper, cucumber, onion, coriander, rice vinegar, salt and pepper. Toss to combine.

2. Fish Fillets: prepare three large, shallow dishes. In the first combine the breadcrumbs, parsley, bran and wheatgerm, tarragon, salt and pepper. In the second, place the flour. In the third, place the egg. Dredge a fish fillet with the flour first, shaking off the excess. Then coat the fillet with egg. Then dredge the fillet with the breadcrumb mixture. Repeat with the rest of the fillets. Place the prepared fillets on a plate lined with waxed paper and set aside.

3. Heat half of the oil in a large non-stick frying pan over a medium-high heat. Add 2 of the fillets and cook, turning once, or until golden brown, about 10 minutes. Repeat with the remaining oil and fillets. Serve topped with Mandarin Salsa.

POULTRY

CHICKEN FRIED RICE (Makes 4 servings)

Chinese fried rice is generally high in fat and low in protein and fibre. This low-Gi version is loaded with chicken and colourful vegetables, and won't leave you feeling hungry again soon after eating it.

180g/6oz brown rice
Pinch salt
350ml/12fl oz chicken stock, made from a cube
1tsp sesame oil
2 boneless skinless chicken breasts (125g/4½oz each), chopped
50g/1¾oz sliced mushrooms
1 spring onion, chopped
2 carrots, diced
1 stick celery, sliced
150g/5oz cooked chickpeas
4tbsp low salt or light soy sauce
125g/4½oz bean sprouts

1. In a saucepan bring the rice, salt and chicken stock to boil. Reduce the heat to low, cover and cook for about 25 minutes or until the liquid is absorbed. Fluff with a fork and set aside.

2. In a large, non-stick frying pan heat the oil over a medium-high heat. Cook the chicken and mushrooms for about 8 minutes or until the chicken is no longer pink inside. Add the onions, carrot, celery, chickpeas and cooked rice. Cook, stirring, for 2 minutes to combine.

3. Add the remaining chicken stock and soy sauce and cook for 5 minutes. Add the bean sprouts and toss to combine.

Vegetarian variation: substitute vegetable stock for the chicken stock and 1/2 cup chopped firm tofu for the chicken.

CHICKEN CURRY (Makes 2 servings)

Vegetable oil cooking spray (ideally olive oil)
1 medium onion, sliced
1tsp curry powder, or more to taste
1 medium carrot, chopped
1 stick celery, sliced
100g/3½oz basmati rice
1 medium apple, chopped
2tbsp raisins
2 boneless, skinless chicken breasts (125g/4½oz each), cooked

1. Spray the oil in a non-stick frying pan, then place it over medium heat. Add the onion and curry powder, stir to coat the onion with the curry, then sauté for 1 minute.

2. Add the carrots and celery, stir to mix, then sauté for 1 minute.

3. Add the rice, apple, raisins and 250 ml/9fl oz of water and stir to mix. Cover the frying pan and let the curry simmer until all of the liquid is absorbed.

4. Add the cooked chicken and heat through for 2 minutes.

CHICKEN SCHNITZEL (Makes 4 servings)

Kids love this dish. You can substitute more traditional veal scaloppini for the chicken.

4 boneless, skinless chicken breasts (125g/4 ¹⁄₂oz each)
60g/2³⁄₄oz wholemeal flour
¹⁄₂tsp freshly ground pepper
2 free range egg whites
20g/³⁄₄oz wheat bran
4tbsp wheatgerm
4tbsp dry wholemeal breadcrumbs
1tsp grated orange zest
1tbsp olive oil
125ml/4 ¹⁄₂fl oz orange juice
125ml/4 ¹⁄₂fl oz chicken stock, made with a cube
75g/3oz dried apricots, thinly sliced
3 spring onions, chopped

1. Using a meat mallet or rolling pin, pound the chicken breasts between 2 pieces of non-stick baking parchment until about 5mm/¹⁄₄ in thick.

2. In a large shallow dish or pie plate combine the flour and pepper. In another shallow dish or pie plate, whisk the egg whites. In a third dish or pie plate combine the bran, wheatgerm, breadcrumbs and orange zest.

3. Pat the chicken dry and dredge in the flour mixture, shaking off any excess. Dip in egg white, letting the excess drip off, then dredge in the bran mixture, coating completely.

4. In a large non-stick frying pan, heat the oil over a medium-high heat. Fry the chicken (in batches if necessary) for 4 minutes on each side or until golden brown and just cooked through. Transfer to a platter and place in a warm oven.

5. In the same frying pan, combine the orange juice, stock and apricots. Bring to the boil and allow to reduce until slightly thickened and syrupy, about 3 minutes. Stir in the spring onion. Pour the sauce over the chicken and serve.

CHICKEN JAMBALAYA (Makes 4 servings)

Jambalaya is a traditional Cajun dish in which rice is used to sop up the rich juices of the stew.

2tsp vegetable oil
2 sticks celery, chopped
2 cloves garlic, crushed
1 onion, chopped
500g/1lb 2oz boneless, skinless chicken breasts, cut into 1cm/½in cubes
2tsp dried thyme
2tsp dried oregano
1tsp chilli powder or to taste

¼tsp cayenne pepper (optional)
500ml/18fl oz chicken stock, made with a cube
2 green peppers, seeded and diced
2x410g cans chopped tomatoes
1x410g can red kidney beans, drained and rinsed
150g/5oz brown rice
1 bay leaf
4tbsp chopped fresh flat-leaf parsley

1. Heat the oil in a Dutch oven or cast iron casserole over medium-high heat. Add the celery, garlic and onion and cook until the onion has softened, about 5 minutes. Add the chicken, thyme, oregano, chilli powder and cayenne pepper and cook, stirring, for 5 minutes.

2. Add the chicken stock, green peppers, tomatoes, kidney beans, rice and bay leaf, and bring to a boil. Reduce the heat to low, cover and simmer, stirring occasionally, for about 35 minutes or until the rice is tender. Let the dish stand for 5 minutes. Remove the bay leaf and discard. Stir in the parsley before serving.

ORANGE CHICKEN WITH ALMONDS (Makes 2 servings)

Fans of sweet-and-sour dishes will enjoy this orange-flavoured chicken. The almonds add calcium. Serve over basmati rice.

2 oranges
1tbsp vegetable oil
2 boneless skinless, chicken breasts (125g/4½oz each), diced
2tsp grated fresh ginger
¼tsp freshly ground pepper
2 spring onions, chopped
1 each red and green pepper, seeded and chopped
Pinch hot pepper or chilli flakes
4tbsp chicken stock, made with a cube, or water (add ¼tsp salt if using water)
3tbsp soy sauce
2tsp cornflour
50g/1¾oz sliced almonds, toasted

1. Using a rasp or grater, remove 1tsp of the orange zest and set aside. Cut away the orange zest and pith from 1 of the oranges and discard. Chop the

orange flesh coarsely. Cut the other orange in half and squeeze out the juice; set aside, discarding the rind.

2. In a large non-stick frying pan or wok heat 1 ½tsp of the oil over a medium high heat. Cook the chicken, ginger and a pinch of pepper for about 6 minutes or until the chicken is no longer pink inside. Transfer to a plate. Add the remaining oil to the frying pan and cook the spring onion, red and green pepper, and hot pepper flakes, stirring constantly, for about 6 minutes or until just tender.

3. In a small bowl, whisk together the chicken stock, soy sauce, reserved orange zest and juice, cornflour and remaining pepper. Add the chicken, chopped orange and vegetable mixture to the frying pan and cook, stirring, for about 5 minutes or until the sauce is thickened and the chicken and vegetables are coated. Sprinkle with almonds and serve with rice.

CHICKEN TARRAGON WITH MUSHROOMS
(Makes 2 servings)

Tarragon adds a light French flavour. The variation below is great for entertaining.

2tsp vegetable oil
2 boneless, skinless chicken breasts (125g/4¹⁄₂oz each)
Freshly ground pepper
1tsp soft margarine
1 small onion, chopped
250g/9oz mushrooms sliced
3tbsp vermouth or white wine
1tbsp chopped fresh tarragon
125ml/4 ¹⁄₂oz chicken stock or water

1 Heat the oil in a non-stick frying pan over a medium-high heat. Sprinkle the chicken with fresh pepper and sauté for about 6 minutes on each side until no longer pink inside. Transfer to a plate and cover to keep warm.

2 In the same pan add the margarine and sauté the onion and mushrooms, stirring constantly, until soft, about 5 minutes. Add the vermouth and tarragon and simmer for 1 minute. Add the stock and simmer for 2 minutes until reduced by half. Season with pepper. Serve the sauce over the chicken.

SPICY ROASTED CHICKEN WITH TOMATOES AND TARRAGON (Makes 4 servings)

This recipe is from our friend Meryle. Serve it with basmati rice or quinoa to soak up the sauce.

250g/9oz cherry tomatoes, halved
5 cloves garlic, crushed
4tbsp extra virgin olive oil
2tbsp chopped fresh tarragon
½-1tsp red pepper or chilli flakes or to taste
4 boneless, skinless chicken breasts (125g/4½oz each)
1tsp each salt and freshly ground pepper

1. Preheat the oven to 220°C, Gas 7.

2. In a large bowl toss the tomatoes with the garlic, oil, 1 tbsp of the tarragon, and red pepper flakes.

3. Place the tomatoes in a shallow roasting pan in a single layer around the chicken. Sprinkle the chicken and tomato mixture with salt and pepper. Roast for 30 to 35 minutes or until the chicken is no longer pink inside. Transfer the chicken to a platter. Spoon the tomatoes and juices over the chicken and sprinkle with remaining tarragon.

ZESTY BARBECUED CHICKEN (Makes 4 servings)

The marinade in this recipe helps keep the breasts moist when they are cooked.

4tbsp lemon juice
2tsp chopped fresh rosemary
2tsp vegetable oil
4 boneless, skinless chicken breasts (125g/4 ½oz each)
Quarter of Zesty Barbecue Sauce (see right)

1. In a bowl whisk together the lemon juice, rosemary and oil. Add the chicken breasts; toss to coat. Marinate at room temperature for 30 minutes.

2. Preheat an oiled grill to medium-high.

3. Remove the chicken from marinade (discarding the marinade) and brush with Zesty Barbecue Sauce; grill for 6 minutes. Turn, brush with more sauce and grill for another 6 minutes or until the chicken is no longer pink inside.

ZESTY BARBECUE SAUCE (Makes about 375ml/12fl oz)

This sauce will keep up to 2 weeks chilled in an airtight container.

1x500g carton sieved tomatoes or sugocasa
2 cloves garlic, crushed
4tbsp quality apple juice
4tbsp tomato puree
2tbsp cider vinegar
1tbsp Splenda
1tbsp Dijon mustard
1tsp chilli powder or to taste (mild or medium strength)
½tsp Worcestershire sauce
¼tsp each salt and freshly ground pepper

1. In a large saucepan combine the tomato sauce, garlic, apple juice, tomato puree, vinegar, Splenda, mustard, chilli powder, Worcestershire sauce, salt and pepper; bring to boil. Reduce heat and simmer uncovered for about 20 minutes or until reduced and thickened.

MEAT
MEATLOAF (Makes 6 servings)

700g/1lb 9oz extra-lean minced beef
250ml/9fl oz tomato juice
75g/3oz large flake oats
1 egg, lightly beaten
1 medium onion, chopped
1tbsp Worcestershire sauce
½tsp salt (optional)
¼tsp freshly ground pepper

1. Preheat the oven to 180°C, Gas 4.

2. In a large bowl combine all ingredients. Mix lightly but thoroughly.

3. Press the meatloaf mixture into a 20 x 10cm/8 x 4in loaf pan. Bake for 1 hour until firm when pressed, or until a meat thermometer inserted into the centre registers 70°C. Let the meat loaf stand for 5 minutes before draining off any juices and slicing it.

HORSERADISH BURGERS (Makes 4 servings)

The combination of beef and horseradish makes these burgers a hit with meat lovers. For a spicier horseradish flavour, simply smother the top with some more horseradish.

1 small onion, grated
1 clove garlic, minced
2tbsp horseradish
2tbsp brown or steak sauce
1tbsp Dijon mustard
1tbsp Worcestershire sauce
2tbsp chopped fresh oregano
¼tsp salt

½tsp freshly ground pepper
2tbsp wheat bran
2tbsp wheatgerm
450g/1lb extra-lean minced beef
2 wholemeal baps, halved
4 leaves lettuce
1 tomato, sliced
4tbsp alfalfa sprouts (optional)

1. In a large bowl stir together the onion, garlic, horseradish, sauce, mustard, Worcestershire sauce, oregano, salt and pepper. Mix in the bran and wheatgerm. Let it stand for 5 minutes. Using your hands, mix in the beef until the mixture is well combined.

2. Preheat an oiled grill. Form the meat mixture into 4 patties about 1cm/1/2 inch thick. Place on a grill or in a non-stick frying pan and grill or cook, turning once, for about 12 minutes, or until no longer pink inside. Place the patties on each half of the baps. Top with lettuce, tomato slices and sprouts (if using).

BEEF AND AUBERGINE CHILLI (Makes 4 servings)

The addition of aubergine gives this chili a delicious twist. Sprinkle with low-fat Cheddar cheese for extra zip.

350g/12oz lean minced beef
1tbsp vegetable oil
2 onions, chopped
4 cloves garlic, crushed
1tsp chilli powder or to taste, mild or hot
1tbsp dried oregano
1tsp ground cumin

2 green peppers, seeded and chopped
1 medium aubergine, chopped
2x410g cans chopped tomatoes
75g/3oz tomato puree
1x410g can red kidney beans, drained and rinsed

1. In a large saucepan over a medium-high heat brown the beef, stirring until crumbly, and remove to a plate. In the same saucepan heat the oil over a medium heat and add the onions, garlic, chilli powder, oregano and cumin, stirring for about 5 minutes or until softened.

2. Add the peppers and aubergine; cook for 10 minutes or until the aubergine is lightly golden. Add the tomatoes, tomato puree and browned beef; bring to

the boil. Reduce the heat and add the beans. Simmer for about 1 hour or until the aubergine is very tender.

RIGATONI WITH MINI-MEATBALLS
(Makes 4 to 6 servings)

For busy families, a little meal preplanning always helps during the week. This hearty casserole can be made ahead of time and frozen for another day.

250g/9oz minced turkey
2tbsp chopped fresh flat-leaf parsley
1 large clove garlic, crushed
½tsp salt
Pinch freshly ground pepper
1tbsp extra virgin olive oil
1 onion, chopped
1 small aubergine, chopped
1 courgette, chopped
1 small carrot, finely chopped
1tbsp dried oregano
1 litre/1 ¾ pint puréed tomatoes e.g. sugocasa, passata etc
½x410g can red kidney beans, drained
300g/10oz rigatoni pasta
2tbsp grated Parmesan cheese

1. Preheat oven to 180°C, Gas 4.

2. In a bowl mix together the chicken, parsley, garlic, pinch of the salt and pepper until well combined. Using wet hands, roll 1 rounded tsp of the mixture into a small meatball and place on a baking sheet lined with non-stick baking parchment. Repeat with the remaining mixture. Bake for about 8 minutes or until no longer pink inside.

3. Meanwhile in a large saucepan heat the oil over medium-high heat. Cook the onion and aubergine for about 8 minutes or until golden and softened. Reduce the heat to medium and add the courgette, carrot and oregano. Cook, stirring, for about 5 minutes or until softened. Add the puréed tomatoes and remaining salt; bring to the boil. Add the cooked meatballs and beans; reduce the heat and simmer for about 30 minutes or until the sauce is slightly thickened.

4. Meanwhile in a large pot of boiling salted water cook the rigatoni for about 10 minutes or until al dente. Drain and add to the meatballs and sauce; stir to combine. Sprinkle with Parmesan cheese.

PORK MEDALLIONS DIJON (Makes 6 servings)

Eating the green-light way doesn't mean you have to sacrifice flavour. This pork is fork tender, and the tasty sauce is rich and creamy.

2 pork tenderloins (about 350g/12oz each)
5tbsp wholemeal flour
¾tsp each salt and freshly ground pepper
2tbsp olive oil
2 onions, thinly sliced
1 clove garlic, crushed
¼ cup Dijon mustard
300ml/½ pint skimmed milk
125ml/4 ½ fl oz dry white wine
1tbsp chopped fresh tarragon

1. Slice the pork into 2cm/¾in medallions. Place between 2 pieces of non-stick baking parchment and, using a meat mallet or rolling pin, pound to about 5mm/¼in thickness.

2. On a dinner plate combine 3tbsp of the flour and ½tsp each of the salt and pepper; dredge the pork. In a large non-stick frying pan heat 1tbsp of the oil over a medium-high heat. Cook the pork until golden brown on both sides, 5 to 7 minutes; transfer to a plate and cover to keep warm.

3. In the same frying pan heat the remaining oil over a medium heat. Cook the onions and garlic, stirring often, for 5 minutes or until softened. Reduce heat to medium-low; cook, stirring occasionally, for 10 minutes or until golden. Add the remaining flour and stir to coat the onion. Add the mustard; cook for 2 minutes.

Stir in the milk, wine and the remaining salt and pepper. Cook, stirring constantly, until thickened. If the mixture is too thick, stir in 1 tbsp warm water then stir in the tarragon. Return the pork to the pan and cook until heated through, about 1 minute.

MUSHROOM AND GRAVY PORK CHOPS
Makes 4 servings)

Nothing turns food into comfort food better than gravy. For a change, substitute chicken for pork chops.

1tsp Italian seasoning
½tsp dried basil
½tsp freshly ground pepper
4 boneless pork loin chops, about 150g/5oz each
2tsp extra virgin olive oil
1 large onion, thinly sliced
500g/1lb 2oz mushrooms, sliced
1tbsp chopped fresh thyme
2tbsp wholemeal flour
250ml/9fl oz chicken stock, from a cube

1. In a small bowl combine the Italian seasoning, basil and ¼tsp pepper. Sprinkle evenly on both sides of the pork chops.

2. In a large non-stick frying pan heat the oil over a medium-high heat. Brown the chops on both sides; transfer to a plate and cover to keep warm. Add the onion, mushrooms, thyme and remaining pepper to the pan. Cook, stirring, for 10 minutes. Sprinkle with flour and cook, stirring, for 1 minute.

3. Pour in the stock, stirring to combine, and bring to the boil. Reduce the heat and simmer for about 3 minutes or until slightly thickened. Return the pork chops to the frying pan and cook, turning occasionally, for about 5 minutes or until just a hint of pink remains inside the pork.

PORK TENDERLOIN WITH APPLE COMPOTE

(Makes 3 servings)

Serve this comforting dish with Brussels sprouts, sliced carrots and some boiled new potatoes tossed in lemon juice and parsley.

1tbsp Dijon mustard
½tsp dried sage
¼tsp dried thyme
Pinch each salt and freshly ground pepper
1 pork tenderloin (about 350g/12oz)
1tbsp vegetable oil
Apple Compote:
1tsp vegetable oil
2 small apples, cored and diced
1 onion, finely chopped
¼tsp dried thyme
Pinch each salt and pepper
2tbsp currants
2tbsp apple juice

1. Preheat the oven to 200°C, Gas 6.

2. In a small bowl stir together the mustard, sage, thyme, salt and pepper. Rub the mixture all over tenderloin.

3. In an ovenproof non-stick frying pan heat 1tbsp of oil over a medium-high heat. Brown the tenderloin on one side, turn over and place the frying pan in the oven for about 20 minutes or until the pork has only a hint of pink inside. Let stand for 5 minutes before slicing.

4. Apple Compote: meanwhile in another non-stick frying pan heat 1tsp oil over a medium-high heat. Cook the apples, onion, thyme, salt and pepper for 5 minutes or until light golden. Add the currants and apple juice; cook for 1 minute or until the apples are just tender. Slice the tenderloin and serve with the Apple Compote.

SNACKS

CRUNCHY CHICKPEAS (Makes at least 8 servings)

2x410g cans chickpeas, drained and rinsed
2tbsp extra virgin olive oil or vegetable oil
½tsp salt
Pinch cayenne pepper

1. Preheat the oven to 200°C, Gas 6.

2. In a large bowl, toss the chickpeas with oil, salt and cayenne pepper. Spread on a large baking sheet in a single layer.

3. Bake for about 45 minutes or until golden, shaking the pan a couple of times during cooking. Let cool completely.

Helpful Hint: add more salt or other spices to change the flavour of the chickpeas.

CRANBERRY CINNAMON BRAN MUFFINS
(Makes 12 muffins)

40g/1½oz wheat bran
30g/1oz All-Bran or 100% Bran cereal
¼tsp salt
125ml/4fl oz boiling water
250ml/9fl oz skimmed milk
1x75g pack dried cranberries

5tbsp Splenda
1 free range egg
4tbsp vegetable oil
150g/5oz wholemeal flour
1¼tsp bicarbonate of soda
1tsp ground cinnamon

1. Preheat the oven to 190°C, Gas 5. Line 12 muffin tins with paper or foil liners.

2. In a bowl combine the bran, cereal and salt. Pour boiling water over and stir to combine. Stir in the milk and cranberries and set aside.

3. In another bowl whisk together the Splenda, egg and oil. Stir into the bran mixture.

4. In a large bowl, stir together the flour, baking soda and cinnamon. Pour the bran mixture over the flour mixture and stir until just combined. Divide the batter among the muffin tins. Bake for about 20 minutes or until a tester inserted in the centre comes out clean.

Make Ahead: These muffins can be kept at room temperature for about 2 days or frozen for up to 1 month. (Wrap each muffin individually before freezing to help prevent freezer burn. Then place them in a resealable plastic bag or airtight container.)

CARROT MUFFINS (Makes 12 muffins)

These healthy muffins are a delightful source of fibre.

125g/4 ½oz wholemeal flour
20g/¾oz wheat bran
40g/1 ½oz ground flaxseed
4tbsp Splenda
2tsp baking powder
½tsp bicarbonate soda
2tsp ground cinnamon
1tsp ground ginger
¼tsp salt

1x284ml carton buttermilk
2 medium free range eggs
4tbsp vegetable oil
1tsp vanilla extract
1 large carrot, finely grated
75g/3oz raisins, softened in hot
water for 10 minutes and drained
40g/1 ½oz chopped pecans

1. Preheat the oven to 190°C, Gas 5. Line 12 deep muffin tins with paper or foil liners.

2. In a large bowl combine the flour, bran, flaxseed, Splenda, baking powder, bicarbonate, cinnamon, ginger and salt.

3. In a small bowl whisk together the buttermilk, egg, oil and vanilla. Stir in the carrot, raisins and pecans. Add the flour mixture and stir until just combined.

4. Divide the batter among the muffin tins. Bake for 20 to 25 minutes until firm to touch or until a tester inserted in the centre of the muffin comes out clean.

Make Ahead: see page 181.

APPLE BRAN MUFFINS (Makes 12 muffins)

Ruth created this recipe several years ago when I was trying to lose weight. We would make large batches and freeze them. Then, whenever I needed a snack, I'd warm one in the microwave. They were so convenient and delicious.

45g/1 ½oz All-Bran or Bran Buds
cereal
250ml/9fl oz skimmed milk
100g/3 ½oz wholemeal flour
15g/½oz Splenda
2tsp baking powder
½tsp bicarbonate of soda
¼tsp salt
1tsp ground allspice

½tsp ground cloves
180g/6oz oat bran
100g/3 ½oz raisins
1 large apple, peeled and cut into
5mm/¼-inch cubes
1 free range omega-3 egg, lightly
beaten
2 tsp vegetable oil
150g/5oz apple sauce (unsweetened)

1. Preheat the oven to 180 °C, Gas 4. Line 12 deep muffin tins with paper or foil liners.

2. Mix the cereal and skimmed milk in a bowl and let stand for a few minutes.

3. In a large bowl mix the flour, Splenda, baking powder, bicarbonate, salt, allspice and cloves. Stir in the oat bran, raisins and apple.

4. In a small bowl combine the egg, oil and applesauce. Stir, along with the cereal mixture, into the dry ingredients.

5. Divide the batter among the muffin tins. Bake until lightly browned, about 20 minutes.

Make Ahead: See page 181.

WHOLEMEAL FRUIT SCONES (Makes 8 scones)

Enjoy these scones with a hot cup of tea. They are even better with a little sugar-free fruit spread.

180g/6oz wholemeal flour
75g/3oz oat bran
75g/3oz chopped dried apricots or dried cranberries
2tbsp Splenda
2tsp baking powder
½tsp salt
¼tsp nutmeg
4tbsp soft margarine
160ml/5 ½fl oz skimmed milk
½ free range medium egg, beaten

1. Preheat the oven to 220 °C, Gas 7.

2. In a large bowl combine the flour, oat bran, dried apricots or cranberries, Splenda, baking powder, salt and nutmeg. Using your fingers, rub the margarine into the flour mixture to combine. Add the milk and stir lightly with a fork to form a soft dough.

3. Place the dough on a floured surface and knead gently about 5 times. Pat the dough out to 1cm/½ in thickness. Cut the dough into 8 squares, or use cookie or biscuit cutter to cut out rounds. Place on a non-stick baking sheet and brush the tops with beaten egg. Bake for about 12 minutes or until golden on the bottom and firm when pressed.

STRAWBERRY TEA BREAD

(Makes 2 loaves, with 14 to 16 slices each. One serving is 1 slice)

This recipe makes two loaves, one for now and one for the freezer. A slice makes a perfect snack or delicious dessert paired with sliced berries.

250g/9oz wholemeal flour
150g/5oz porridge oats
20g/³⁄₄oz wheat bran
1tsp ground cinnamon
1tsp bicarbonate of soda
½tsp baking powder
½tsp salt
3 medium free range eggs, beaten
12tbsp Splenda
125ml/4 ½fl oz vegetable oil
125ml/4 ½fl oz skimmed milk
1tsp vanilla extract
500g/1lb 2oz strawberries, fresh or frozen and thawed, mashed

1. Preheat the oven to 190°C, Gas 5. Oil two 23 x13 cm/9 x 5 in loaf tins (1kg/2lb size).

2. In a large bowl stir together the flour, oats, bran, cinnamon, bicarbonate, baking powder and salt; set aside.

3. In a separate bowl whisk together the eggs, Splenda, oil, milk and vanilla. Pour over the dry ingredients and stir just until moistened. Stir in the strawberries.

4. Divide mixture evenly between the pans. Bake for 45 to 50 minutes or until a cake tester inserted in the centre comes out clean. Let cool in the pan on a rack for 15 minutes. Turn out on to a rack and let cool completely.

Make Ahead: wrap in cling film or foil and store at room temperature up to 3 days, or wrap in cling film and heavy-duty foil and freeze up to 1 month.

DESERTS
BERRY CRUMBLE (Makes 6 servings)

This is one of Ruth's favourite green-light desserts. Though it's best made with fresh berries during the summer, it's also lovely with frozen fruit.

750g/1lb 10oz fresh or frozen berries, such as raspberries, blackberries, blueberries and sliced strawberries
1 large apple, cored and chopped
2tbsp wholemeal flour
1–2tbsp Splenda
½tsp ground cinnamon
Topping:
90g/3 ¼oz jumbo oats
50g/1 ¾oz chopped pecans or walnuts
3tbsp Splenda
1tbsp brown sugar
4tbsp soft margarine, melted
1tsp ground cinnamon

1. Preheat the oven to 180°C, Gas 4.

2. In a 20cm/8 in square baking dish combine the berries and apple.

3. In a separate bowl, combine the flour Splenda and cinnamon. Sprinkle over the fruit and toss gently.

4. Topping: in a medium bowl combine the oats, pecans, Splenda, brown sugar, margarine and cinnamon. Sprinkle over fruit mixture. Bake for about 30 minutes or until the fruit is tender and the top is golden.

Variation: prepare as above and microwave on high for about 6 minutes or until the fruit is tender. The top won't get golden or crisp in the microwave.

PLUM CRUMBLE (Makes 6 servings)

Crumbles are an ideal green-light dessert and can be made with a wide array of fruit.

Try using pears instead of the plums, cutting back slightly on the amount of Splenda.

800g/1 ½lb ripe plums, halved and pitted
1tbsp Splenda
1tbsp cornflour
½tsp ground ginger
½tsp ground cinnamon
Topping:
75g/3oz large flake oats
60g/2 ¾oz wholemeal flour
3tbsp Splenda
1tbsp brown sugar
50g/1 ¾oz chopped almonds or pecans
4tbsp soft margarine
1tsp grated orange zest
½tsp ground cinnamon
¼tsp ground cardamom

1. Preheat the oven to 180°C, Gas 4.

2. In a bowl toss the plums with Splenda, cornflour, ginger and cinnamon. Arrange evenly in a deep 23 cm/9 in pie plate.

3. Topping: in a bowl combine the oats, flour, Splenda, brown sugar, almonds, margarine, orange zest, cinnamon and cardamom. Using your fingers, rub the ingredients together to a crumbly dough. Sprinkle evenly over the fruit mixture. Bake for 35 to 40 minutes or until topping is golden and fruit mixture is bubbling.

Make Ahead: chill for up to 2 days.

APPLE RASPBERRY COFFEE CAKE (Makes 9 servings)

A piece of this fruit-laden cake makes a delectable light dessert. It can be refrigerated for up to 3 days.

125g/4 ½oz wholemeal flour
20g/³/₄oz wheat bran
8tbsp Splenda
1½tsp baking powder
½tsp bicarbonate of soda
¼tsp ground cinnamon
¼tsp ground nutmeg
Pinch salt
125ml/4 ½fl oz buttermilk
4tbsp soft margarine, melted and cooled
1 medium free range egg, beaten
2tsp vanilla extract
125g/4 ½oz fresh raspberries
1 apple, cored and diced
Topping:
30g/1 ¼oz cup jumbo oats
3tbsp Splenda
1tbsp brown sugar
2tbsp chopped pecans
1tbsp soft margarine

1. Preheat the oven to 180°C, Gas 4. Line base of a 20cm/8in square shallow cake tin with non-stick baking parchment.

2. In a large bowl whisk together the flour, bran, Splenda, baking powder, bicarbonate, cinnamon, nutmeg and salt; set aside.

3. In another bowl whisk together the buttermilk, margarine, egg and vanilla. Pour over the flour mixture and stir until moistened. Spread two thirds of the batter in the prepared cake tin.

4. Toss the raspberries and apple together and sprinkle over the batter. Dollop with the remaining batter, smoothing gently with wet spatula.

5. Topping: in a bowl mix together the oats, Splenda, brown sugar, pecans and margarine until combined. Sprinkle over the top of the cake; press gently into the batter. Bake for about 30 minutes or until a tester inserted in the centre comes out clean.

ONE-BOWL CHOCOLATE CAKE (Makes 8 servings)

This delicious cake is green-light when served with fresh berries. You can make a yellow light version with chocolate ganache icing for a special occasion (see Variation below).

Vegetable oil, to grease
200g/7oz wholemeal flour
12tbsp Splenda
35g/1 ¼oz unsweetened cocoa powder
1 ½tsp bicarbonate of soda
1 ½tsp baking powder
½tsp salt

1 free range egg
1 egg white
160ml/5 ¾fl oz buttermilk
125g/4 ½ oz apple sauce
2tbsp vegetable oil
1tsp vanilla extract
Grated zest of 1 orange

1. Preheat the oven to 180°C, Gas 4. Oil a 20 cm/8 in round deep cake tin or spring form pan. Cut a round of baking parchment and line bottom of the tin.

2. In a mixer, food processor or blender mix together all ingredients just until smooth.

3. Pour the batter into a prepared tin, smoothing the top. Bake for 20 to 25 minutes or until the top springs back when lightly touched and a cake tester inserted in the centre comes out clean.

4. Cool in the tin on a rack for 30 minutes. Turn out from the tin and remove the paper; allow to cool completely on a rack.

Ganache variation: melt 225g/8oz of 70% chocolate in a bowl set over barely simmering water. Remove from the heat and whisk in 300ml/1.2 pint low-fat soy milk until smooth. Cool and beat again before using. Spread the ganache over the top and sides of cake.

APPLE PIE COOKIES
(Makes about 18 cookies. One serving is one cookie)

These cookies combine all the flavours of traditional apple pie and have a texture like a soft granola bar. A great snack.

100g/3 ½oz large flake oats
90g/3oz wholemeal flour
1tsp ground cinnamon
½tsp baking powder
Pinch each nutmeg and salt

200g/7oz apple sauce
5tbsp Splenda
1 medium free range egg, beaten
2tsp vanilla extract
1 apple, cored and finely diced

1. Preheat the oven to 140°C, Gas 1. Line a baking sheet with non-stick baking parchment.

2. In a large bowl combine the oats, flour, cinnamon, baking powder, nutmeg and salt.

3. In a separate bowl whisk together the apple sauce, Splenda, egg and vanilla. Pour over the oat mixture and stir to combine. Add the apple and stir to distribute evenly.

4. Drop by heaping tablespoonfuls on to a prepared baking sheet. Bake for about 25 minutes or until firm and lightly golden. Let cool completely.

Make Ahead: keep in airtight container for up to 3 days or freeze for up to 2 weeks.

PECAN BROWNIES
(Makes 16 brownies. One serving is one brownie)

Brownies, you ask? That's right. These are packed with fibre and are absolutely scrumptious, so get baking!

1x410g can white or red kidney, or black beans, drained and rinsed
125ml/4½fl oz skimmed milk
1 medium free range egg, beaten
4tbsp soft margarine, melted
1tbsp vanilla extract
12tbsp Splenda
60g/2 ¾oz wholemeal flour
60g/2 ¾oz unsweetened cocoa powder
1tsp baking powder
Pinch salt
50g/1 ¾oz chopped toasted pecans

1. Preheat the oven to 180°C, Gas 4. Line a 20cm/8 in square cake tin with non-stick baking parchment.

2. In a food processor purée the beans until coarse. Add the milk, egg, margarine and vanilla and purée until smooth, scraping down the sides a few times. Set aside.

3. In a large bowl combine Splenda, flour, cocoa, baking powder and salt. Pour the bean mixture over flour mixture. Stir to combine. Scrape the batter into a prepared pan, smoothing the top. Sprinkle with pecans.

4. Bake for about 18 minutes or until a cake tester inserted in the centre comes out clean. Let cool on a rack, then cut into 16 squares.

Make Ahead: wrap the brownies in plastic wrap or store in an airtight container for up to 4 days. They can also be frozen for up to 2 weeks.

CREAMY LEMON SQUARES
(Makes 36 squares. One serving is 2 squares)

These tiny treats make an ideal mid-afternoon pick-me-up.

60g/2¾oz wholemeal flour
20g/¾oz wheat bran
4tbsp ground almonds
4tbsp Splenda
4tbsp soft margarine
Filling:
16tbsp Splenda
3 medium free range eggs, beaten
2tsp grated lemon zest
125ml/4 ½fl oz fresh lemon juice
4tbsp buttermilk
2tsp cornflour
1tsp baking powder

1. Preheat the oven to 180°C, Gas 4. Lightly oil a 20cm/8in square cake tin.

2. In a mixer or food processor combine the flour, bran, almonds and Splenda. Cut in the margarine until the mixture is crumbly.

3. Press the mixture evenly into the bottom of a prepared baking pan. Bake for 20 to 25 minutes or until lightly browned. Set aside to cool, leaving the oven on.

4. Filling: in a bowl whisk together the Splenda and egg. Stir in lemon zest and juice, buttermilk, zest, cornflour and baking powder. Pour over the baked base and return to the oven for 15 to 20 minutes or until the filling is set. Let cool to room temperature, then chill for at least 2 hours before cutting into squares.

Make Ahead: store in airtight container up to 3 days or freeze up to 1 month.

APPENDIX
COMPLETE Gi DIET FOOD GUIDE

RED

BEANS

Broad

BEANS (TINNED)

Baked beans with pork

Refried beans

YELLOW

GREEN

BEANS

Black	Lima
Black eyed	Mung
Butter	Pigeon
Chickpeas	Pinto
Haricot/Navy	Romano
Italian	Soy
Kidney	Split
Lentils	

BEANS (TINNED)

Baked beans (low-fat)

Mixed salad beans

Most varieties

Vegetarian chilli

BEVERAGES

Alcoholic drinks
Coconut milk
(Fizzy) drinks
Milk (whole)
Regular coffee
Regular soft drinks
Buttermilk
Sweetened fruit juice

BEVERAGES

Diet soft drinks (caffeinated)
Milk (semi-skimmed)
Red wine
Unsweetened fruit juices:
Apple
Cranberry
Grapefruit
Orange
Pear
Pineapple
Vegetable juice cocktails (e.g. V8)

BEVERAGES

Bottled water
Decaffeinated coffee (with skimmed milk, no sugar)
Diet soft drinks (no caffeine)
Herbal teas
Light instant chocolate
Milk (skimmed)
Soya milk (low-fat, plain)
Tea (with skimmed milk, no sugar)

BREADS

100% stone-ground
wholemeal*

Homemade muffins
(see pages 181-2)

Wholegrain, high-fibre
breads (2½ to 3g of fibre per slice)*

Crispbreads (high-fibre)*

*Limit portions. See p.17

BREADS

Crispbread with fibre

Pitta (wholemeal)

Wholegrain breads

BREADS

Bagels

Baguettes/Croissants

Cereal/Granola bars

Crispbreads

Doughnuts

Hamburger buns

Hot dog buns

Kaiser rolls

Melba toast

Muffins

Pancakes/Waffles

Pizza

Stuffing

Tortillas

White bread

CEREALS

All cold cereals except those listed as yellow or green-light

Granola

Instant/quick-cook porridge oats

Millet

Muesli (commercial)

CEREAL GRAINS

Almond flour

Amaranth

Couscous

Croutons

Millet

Polenta

Rice (short-grain, white, instant)

Rice cakes

Rice noodles

CEREALS

Shredded Wheat Bran

CEREAL GRAINS

Corn

Corn flour

Spelt

Wholemeal Couscous

CEREALS

All-Bran

Alpen Crunchy Bran

High-Fibre Bran

Oat bran

Porridge oats (traditional large-flake e.g. Jordan's)

100% Bran

Soya Protein Powder

Steel-cut oats

CEREAL GRAINS

Arrowroot flour

Barley

Buckwheat Bulgur

Bulgur

Gram flour

Kamut (not puffed)

Kasha (toasted buckwheat)

Quinoa

Rice (basmati, wild, brown, long-grain)

Soya Protein Powder

Wheat berries

Wheatgrain

CONDIMENTS/SEASONINGS

Croutons
Ketchup
Mayonnaise
Tartar sauce

CONDIMENTS/SEASONINGS

Mayonnaise (light)

CONDIMENTS/SEASONINGS

Chilli powder
Extracts (Vanilla etc.)
Flavoured vinegars/sauces
Garlic
Herbs/Spices
Horseradish
Hummus
Lemon/lime juice
Mayonnaise (fat free)
Mustard
Peppers (all types)
Salsa (low sugar)
Soy sauce (low sodium)
Teriyaki sauce
Worcestershire sauce

DAIRY

- Almond milk
- Cheese ~~
- Chocolate milk
- Cottage cheese (regular)
- Cream
- Cream cheese
- Evaporated milk
- Goats' milk
- Light milk
- Soya cream
- Yogurt (regular)
- Yogurt (low-fat)

DAIRY

- Cheese (low fat)
- Cream cheese (light)
- Crème fraîche (low fat)
- Ice cream (low fat)
- Frozen yogurt (low fat, low sugar)
- Milk (semi-skimmed)
- Soft margarine (non-hydrogenated)
- Sour cream (light)
- Sour cream (fat-free)

DAIRY

- Almond milk (low fat)
- Buttermilk (skimmed low fat)
- Cheese (fat free)
- Cottage cheese (low fat or fat free)
- Fruit yogurt (fat free/with sweetener)
- Ice cream (low fat and no added sugar, e.g. Wall's Soft Scoop Light)
- Milk (skimmed)
- Laughing Cow cheese (light)
- Boursin cheese (light)
- Soy cheese (low fat)
- Soya milk (plain, low fat)
- Soy/whey protein powder

FATS/OILS/DRESSINGS

Butter
Coconut oil
Hard margarine
Lard
Mayonnaise
Palm oil
Peanut butter (regular and light)
Salad dressings (regular)
Tropical oils
Vegetable shortening

Limit portion size

FATS/OILS/DRESSINGS

Corn oil
Mayonnaise (light)
Most nuts
100% Peanut butter*
Peanut oil
Salad dressings (light)
Sesame oil
Soft margarine (non-hydrogenated)
Soy oil
Sunflower oil
Vegetable oils

FATS/OILS/DRESSINGS

Flax seed oil*
Mayonnaise (low-fat/low sugar)
Olive oil*
Rapeseed oil*
Salad dressings (low fat/low sugar)
Soft margarine (non-hydrogenated, light)*
Vegetable oil sprays
Vinaigrette

FRUITS – FRESH

Cantaloupe melon
Dates
Honeydew melon
Kumquats
Watermelon

FRUITS – FRESH

Apricots (fresh)
Bananas
Figs
Kiwi
Mangoes
Papaya
Persimmon
Pineapple
Pomegranate

FRUITS – FRESH

Apples
Avocado (¼ per serving)
Blackberries
Blueberries
Cherries
Grapefruit
Grapes
Guavas
Lemons
Limes
Nectarines
Oranges
Peaches
Pears
Plums
Raspberries
Rhubarb
Strawberries

FRUITS – BOTTLED, TINNED, FROZEN, DRIED

All tinned fruit in syrup
Apple purée containing sugar
Most dried fruit*

*For baking, it is OK to use a modest amount of dried fruit

FRUIT SPREADS

Regular fruit spreads

FRUIT JUICES

Fruit drinks
Sweetened juices
Prune
Watermelon

FRUITS – BOTTLED, TINNED, FROZEN, DRIED

Dried apricots
Dried cranberries
Fruit cocktail in juice
Peaches/pears in syrup
Prunes

FRUIT SPREADS

FRUIT JUICES

Apple (unsweetened)
Cranberry (unsweetened)
Grapefruit (unsweetened)
Orange (unsweetened)
Pear (unsweetened)
Pineapple (unsweetened)

FRUITS – BOTTLED, TINNED, FROZEN, DRIED

Apple sauce (no sugar, e.g. Clearspring Organic)
Apple Purée
Dried apples
Frozen berries
Mandarin oranges
Peaches in juice or water

FRUIT SPREADS

Extra fruit/low-sugar spreads
Fruit as first ingredient

FRUIT JUICES

Eat the fruit rather than drink the juice

MEAT, POULTRY, FISH, EGGS AND SOY

MEAT, POULTRY, FISH, EGGS AND SOY

Chicken/turkey leg
Fish tinned in oil
Flank steak
Lamb (Tenderloin, Centre loin chop)
Minced beef (lean)
Pork (Fore shank, Leg shank, Centre cut, Loin chop)
Sirloin tip
Sirloin steak
Turkey bacon
Whole omega-3 eggs (e.g. Columbus)

MEAT, POULTRY, FISH, EGGS AND SOY

All seafood, fresh, frozen or tinned
Back bacon
Beef (Top round steak, Eye round steak)
Chicken breast (skinless)
Egg whites
Lean deli ham
Minced beef (extra lean)
Pork tenderloin
Quorn
Rabbit
Sashimi
Smoked salmon/trout
Soy/whey protein powder
Tofu
Turkey breast (skinless)
Veal (Cutlet, Rib Roast, Blade steak)
Venison

PASTA

All wheat pasta B...
Gnocchi...
Macaroni and cheese
Noodles (tinned)
Pasta filled with cheese or meat

PASTA SAUCES

Alfredo...
Pesto with added sugar...
Sauce with added oil or cream...

PASTA

Rice noodles

PASTA SAUCES

Sauces with vegetables

PASTA

Capellini
Cellophane noodles (mung bean)
Fettuccine
Linguine
Macaroni
Penne
Rigatoni
Spaghetti
Vermicelli

PASTA SAUCES

Light sauces with or without vegetables (no added sugar)

Bagels
Biscuits
Bread
Chocolates and sweets
Coconuts
Cookies
Crisps/Pretzels
Doughnuts
French fries
Ice cream
Jelly (all varieties)
Mixed dried fruit and nuts
Muffins (commercial)
Peanut butter (regular)
Popcorn (regular)
Raisins
Rice cakes
Sorbet
Tortilla chips

SNACKS

Bananas
Dark chocolate (70% cocoa)*
Ice cream (low fat)
Most nuts*
Peanut butter (100% peanuts)
Popcorn (light, microwaveable)

Limit portions. See p.14

SNACKS

Almonds*
Apple purée (unsweetened)
Canned fruits
Cottage cheese (1% or fat free)
Food bars (12–15g protein; 4–5g fat e.g. Myoplex/ Slim-Fast*)
Fruit yogurt (fat free/ with sweetener)
Hazelnuts*
Homemade muffins (see pages 181–2)
Ice cream (low fat and no added sugar e.g. Wall's Soft Scoop Light)
Marmite**
Most fresh fruit
Most fresh vegetables
Most seeds
Nuts (see fats and oils)*
Soy nuts*
Tinned peaches/pears in juice or water
Vegemite**

Limit portions. See p.14
**Caution: high sodium*

SOUPS

All cream-based soup
Pureed vegetable
Tinned black bean
Tinned green peas
Tinned split pea

SUGAR AND SWEETENERS

Corn syrup
Glucose
Honey
Molasses
Sugar (all types)
Treacle

SOUPS

Tinned chicken noodle
Tinned lentil
Tinned tomato

SUGAR AND SWEETENERS

Fructose
Sugar alcohols

SOUPS

All homemade soups made with green-light ingredients
Chunky bean and vegetable soups (e.g. Baxter's Healthy Choice)

SUGAR AND SWEETENERS

Aspartame
Hermesetas Gold
Splenda
Stevia

TINNED/BOTTLED VEGETABLES

Roasted red peppers
Tinned/bottled vegetables
Tinned tomatoes
Tomato puree

VEGETABLES

- Artichokes
- Beets
- Corn
- Potatoes (boiled)
- Pumpkin
- Squash
- Sweet potatoes
- Yams

VEGETABLES

- Alfalfa sprouts
- Asparagus
- Aubergine
- Beans (green/runner)
- Bok choy
- Broccoli
- Brussels sprouts
- Cabbage
- Capers
- Carrots
- Cauliflower
- Celery
- Collard greens
- Courgettes
- Cucumber
- Fennel
- Kale
- Leeks
- Lettuce
- Mangetout
- Mushrooms
- Mustard greens
- Okra
- Olives
- Onions
- Parsley
- Peas
- Peppers
- Peppers (chillies)
- Pickles
- Potatoes (new/small)
- Radicchio
- Radishes
- Sauerkraut
- Spinach
- Spring onions
- Sugar snap peas
- Swiss chard
- Tomatoes

VEGETABLES

- Broad beans
- French fries
- Hash browns
- Parsnip
- Potatoes (fried/roast)
- Potato
- Swede
- Turnip

Acknowledgments

I owe a special debt to Stacey Cameron at Random House who has edited all six of my books to date. Her help and guidance in bringing order to the mountain of feedback from Clinic participants was invaluable. She truly brought the book to life.

My wife, Ruth, Professor Emeritus at the University of Toronto and an authority on changing behaviours, provided penetrating insights into the emotional and behavioural challenges faced by Clinic members. She was also responsible for the recipe selection as she has been for the entire Gi Diet series. I could not ask for a better partner both professionally and personally.

Index